I Can See Your Heart Beat

A Patient's Guide to the Heart's Electrical System

Written by Jeff Schoeben

Illustrated by Erika McGinnis

Cover Art by Greg Prichard

ISBN: 1461112834
ISBN-13: 9781461112839
Library of Congress Control Number: 2011906267

PREFACE

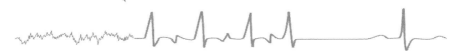

After two decades of assisting numerous doctors while they diagnose and treat the human heart, I felt it was time the general public became more informed about what happens when there is a heart problem. It was, and is, rewarding to help people with blocked arteries, or while they may be in the midst of a heart attack. However, the opportunity to work on the electrical system of the heart was also an inspiration to me to pursue a very satisfying career.

Electrophysiology, the study of the electrical system of the heart, has been around for over 50 years but, to date, there are still patients taking medications who could have a procedure, which would cure the arrhythmia requiring those medications. I have had the opportunity to work with thousands of patients with these curable arrhythmias, and the statement I have heard the most often is, "I wish I had known this procedure was available 20 years ago." These arrhythmias not only effect you, but your family, friends, and co-workers.

I Can See Your Heart Beat is written so you and your family can understand what your arrhythmia is, what happens when it is active, and what can be done to control or cure it. This book will explain the pathway to control and/or cure your arrhythmia, as well as provide insight into what to expect from your doctor and the hospital staff, if you choose to take that path. Moreover, I hope *I Can See Your Heart Beat* stimulates you and your family to ask questions so everyone completely understands what is happening and why. You may hear many new words during explanations of your arrhythmia, so a glossary has been provided in the back of the book with definitions that are, hopefully, easy for you to understand.

A Special Thank You

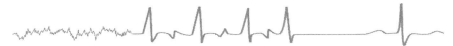

I would like to recognize all the doctors and hospital staff members I have worked with over the years, as they have all had a part in my dedication to patients with heart disease.

A special thanks to my mother, Karen, and my wife, Dawn, who helped edit my thoughts and encouraged me to write this book. My thoughts are also of my children, Derrick and Mallory, who put up with me as I struggled to assemble my observations, experiences, and instincts into words.

TABLE OF CONTENTS

COMMONLY ASKED QUESTIONS:

CHAPTER 1
The Heart

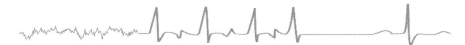

The heart receives information from the brain telling it when to speed up, slow down, or maintain the heart rate. This is accomplished by sending a signal to the SA (sinoatrial) node, which is one of the three natural pacemakers of the heart. The SA node initiates heart rates between 60 and 100 beats per minute. If the SA node is diseased or fails to work, then the AV (atrioventricular) node will provide signals so the heart will beat 40-60 beats per minute. If the SA and AV nodes fail, then the third pacemaker, or ventricular escape rhythm, takes over providing a heart rate of between 20 and 40 beats per minute.

The heart is made up of four chambers: the right and left atria (two upper chambers) and the right and left ventricles (two lower chambers). A membranous tissue called the septum separates the atria and ventricles. Valves separate the upper chambers from the lower chambers. The valve between the right atrium and right ventricle is called the tricuspid valve because it has three leaves. Between the left-sided chambers is the mitral valve, with two leaves. The circulation, or plumbing, of the body is designed, so that blood returning to the heart after giving oxygen to the body, enters the right atrium. Then when the atrium is full, the tricuspid valve opens, allowing the right ventricle to fill with blood. At some point, the tricuspid valve closes due to more pressure in the right ventricle than in the right atrium. Once the pressure of the right ventricle gets high enough, the ventricle contracts, pushing blood through the pulmonary valve toward the lungs. After blood gathers oxygen from the lungs, it drains into the left atrium until the pressure is high enough to open the mitral valve and push the newly oxygenated blood into the left ventricle. Just like in the right ventricle, when the pressure in the left ventricle is high enough, the mitral valve closes and pressure increases in the left ventricle until it is high enough to open the aortic valve, where the ejected blood starts its next trip of providing oxygen to the body. With the plumbing portion of the heart having been explained, let us turn our attention to the electrical part of the heartbeat. (*Figures 1 and 2*)

As the heart develops during pregnancy, it forms a skeleton that separates the four chambers as well as encases the tricuspid and mitral valves. *When the heart develops completely, a heartbeat will start at the sinoatrial node, traveling over the right atrium and over to the left atrium through fibers connecting the upper chambers, down to the junction box between the upper and lower chambers (the AV node). From there it continues through fibers to the tip of the ventricles, spreads out, and a heartbeat occurs.* This is a good spot to focus more in depth about the AV node. (*Figure 3*)

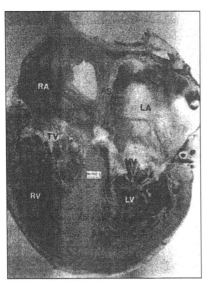

This picture of a dissected heart identifies the right atrium (RA), atrial septum (AS), left atrium (LA), right ventricle (RV), ventricular septum (VS), and left ventricle (LV).

Figure 1

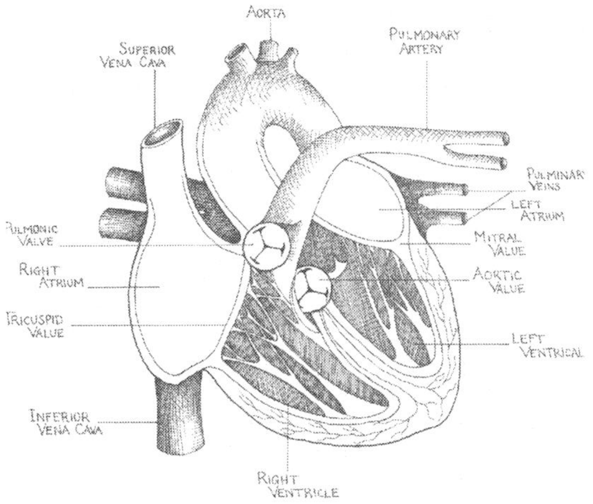

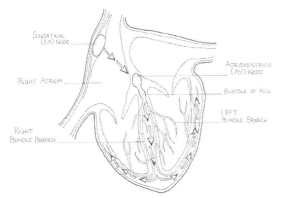

This drawing shows the four chambers of the heart with its valves and connected vessels.

Figure 2

The electrical impulses of the heart begin at the SA (Sinoatrial) node, travel to the AV (Atrio Ventricular) node through the HIS bundle to the bundle branches and, finally, to small fibers after which a heart beat occurs.

Figure 3

The AV node is a regulator for the heart. This means it protects you from high atrial rates continuing to the ventricles. As a rule, the faster the signals at the AV node, the slower it is to let them pass on to the ventricles. An example of this is atrial fibrillation, where heart rates in the upper chambers may be between 350 and 600 beats per minute, but as they reach the AV node, it only allows enough beats through so the heart rate may be 150 beats per minute. This presents a situation that is uncomfortable to a person, but it is not deadly.

NOTES

CHAPTER 2
How Do I Know I Have
An Arrhythmia?

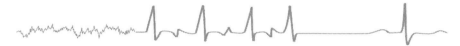

If you are lucky enough to know your family history and you know there is some arrhythmia in your background, when symptoms occur, you will instinctively seek a physician; however, in most instances, with little understanding of what is going on. Others may seek medical attention, saying, "Something just doesn't feel right." When you seek this medical attention, the doctor or nurse will interview you, because they are looking for symptoms to diagnose your problem. Some of these symptoms include, but are not limited to, syncope, near-syncope, palpitations, a flushed feeling, fatigue, shortness of breath, or water retention. Before I review these symptoms, it is important to know these symptoms may also reflect a diagnosis other than an arrhythmia.

Syncope is a medical term for passing out, and near-syncope is almost passing out. Syncope or near-syncope is due to a blood pressure or heart rate problem. If your blood pressure is too low, blood cannot get to the brain and syncope could occur. If syncope is from a heart rate problem, it can be caused by a heart rate, which is too slow or too fast. When the heart rate is too slow, you have good blood flow with each beat, but there are not enough beats to keep oxygen traveling to the brain. The opposite is true for a heart rate, which is too fast: There are enough heartbeats, but they come so quickly, the heart does not have adequate time to fill with blood before the next heartbeat begins.

Another symptom of an arrhythmia diagnosis is palpitations. According to Webster's Dictionary, palpitations are an abnormal rapid or violent beating of the heart. Many of the patients with whom I have worked describe their palpitations as a hard thumping in the chest. There are people who have palpitations or PVCs (premature ventricular contractions) caused by too much caffeine. Usually, reducing caffeine intake will limit or completely stop the palpitations.

Fatigue can be another symptom that leads to an arrhythmia diagnosis. In general, fatigue may be caused by many different variables. You may not be able to work as long or as hard as you used to, or a special activity causes you to tire easily. Fatigue is a vague symptom and needs to be coupled with other symptoms to result in an arrhythmia diagnosis.

Yet another symptom can be a flushed feeling. This will usually occur with minimal activity or at rest. You might describe a situation where you are watching television or reading the newspaper when, suddenly, you get very warm and your face turns red. This happens when the heart rate suddenly rises with normal blood flow. This symptom can last only a few moments or it may last long enough for you to seek medical attention.

Still another symptom can be shortness of breath. Again, this can occur with minimal activity or at rest. Many patients describe a scenario of walking to the mailbox and not being able to catch their breath. Of course, we know the lungs are responsible for breathing, but without the heart, the lungs would not have a job. (*Figure 4*)

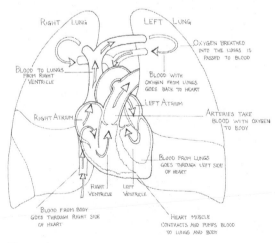

Blood returns from the body to the right side of the heart, and is sent to the lungs to gather oxygen; then the blood is sent to the left side of the heart, where it is sent back out to the body.

Figure 4

The heart pumps blood from the lungs out to the body through arteries and supplies organs, such as the liver and kidneys, and tissues with oxygen, so they may function properly. After the oxygen is used by the body, the blood is returned to the heart through veins, and the deoxygenated blood is pumped through the lungs, where it picks up oxygen and is sent back throughout to the body. (*Figure 5*)

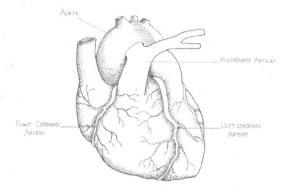

The veins and arteries of the heart are located on the surface, and have branches that go into the muscle, supplying it with oxygen, and returning used blood to the heart to gather more oxygen.

Figure 5

When the body does not function properly, the heart is not always at fault, but sometimes it is a contributing factor effecting the way a specific organ functions. For example, a person notices he/she has swelling in his/her ankles and feet more than usual and may seek a doctor's attention. The doctor or nurse may ask the person if he/she has been urinating less frequently than usual. If so, the swelling may be caused by malfunctioning kidneys leading to water retention. Kidneys may malfunction for a variety of reasons, but family physicians or emergency room doctors will check the heart function to eliminate heart failure as a cause of kidney malfunction.

While these are a few of the symptoms proposing an arrhythmia diagnosis, they may also lead to another diagnosis. Doctors and nurses interview patients to gather as much information or discover as many symptoms as possible to help with a quick and accurate diagnosis. If you experience some of these symptoms and they do not last too long, you may just say, "I'll live with it." While this is one option, as your symptoms progress you will eventually seek help from your family physician, an urgent care center, or an emergency room.

If you have one of the five types of atrial arrhythmias, the symptoms may be short-lived, and you may call your family physician's office during regular office hours to schedule an examination. Alternatively, you may become alarmed by these symptoms, and choose to go to an urgent care center or an emergency room. If you are experiencing these symptoms when you arrive at either the urgent care or the emergency room, the staff will attach a heart monitor or a 12-lead EKG, also called an electrocardiogram, to document your heart's rhythm. Along with evaluating your heart's rhythm, the staff will also take your blood pressure and count your respirations (how many times you breathe per minute).

If the physician you see suspects you have a supraventricular tachycardia (SVT), you will be referred to a cardiologist (a heart doctor). The cardiologist will determine if your heart's rhythm is one that can be managed with medications, or if you will need to see an electrophysiologist, a cardiologist who specializes in the electrical system of the heart. For those with a ventricular arrhythmia, which is a lower-chamber arrhythmia, your choices are limited. Ventricular arrhythmias can be stable or unstable. A stable ventricular arrhythmia is one where you may be a little short of breath, but you have good blood pressure and are fairly comfortable. Unstable ventricular arrhythmias are when you are sweaty, your blood pressure drops, you pass out or come close to passing out. Both atrial, (upper-chamber) and ventricular, (lower-chamber) arrhythmias can be unstable, but an unstable ventricular arrhythmia can be deadly. Unstable ventricular tachycardia and ventricular fibrillation are two heart rhythms that need to be defibrillated (shocked with electricity).

NOTES

CHAPTER 3
You Have Had Symptoms

If your doctor suspects your symptoms are caused by neurocardiogenic syncope, you will be referred to a cardiologist or an electrophysiologist for further evaluation. Neurocardiogenic syncope is an intimidating diagnosis but should not be feared. Neuro relates to the nerves in the body, cardiogenic refers to the heart, and syncope means passing out. There are two basic reasons people become unconscious: one is not enough blood flow or blood pressure, and the other is not enough heart rate. There are nerve receptors that communicate with the heart, letting it know you need a higher heart rate if you are exercising or lower heart rate if you are at rest. These receptors are also responsible for raising or lowering the blood pressure, depending upon the activity. A good example of how the receptors work is getting up out of a chair: When you are sitting, the nerve receptors tell the heart how much blood pressure and at what rate the heart needs to be in order to maintain adequate blood flow to all the vital organs. If you were to stand up quickly, it changes these requirements and you may feel slightly dizzy, until the heart rate and blood pressure are adjusted to accommodate this change in position. With neurocardiogenic syncope, these receptors overreact, telling the heart it is working too hard and to slow down the heart rate or lower the blood pressure, which causes blood to drain from the head and, in turn, causes you to pass out. A simple way to test for neurocardiogenic syncope is a tilt table test. This can be performed by a cardiologist or electrophysiologist and is the least invasive (not putting something into your body) test available. (*Figure* 6)

A tilt table test is an outpatient procedure that will take approximately one hour. Once you enter the procedure room, one of the staff members may or may not start an IV, depending upon which protocol your doctor uses. Next, you will have a 12-lead EKG attached and a blood pressure cuff put on your arm. You will also be strapped to the table for safety, just in case you pass out. Your arms will usually be left free so you can scratch if needed. Once a baseline set of vital signs is taken, the table will be tilted to an 80° angle and another set of vital signs will be taken immediately. If no symptoms occur, the vital signs will be taken every 2 or 3 minutes for a total of 20 to 45 minutes. If symptoms start occurring, the vital signs will be taken repeatedly until a dramatic drop in blood pressure has been demonstrated and documented. The goal of the tilt table is to demonstrate the dramatic drop in blood pressure, but not to allow you to pass out. Once the symptoms are demonstrated, you will be returned to a lying position until you recover. In some protocols, you will stand for 20 minutes, and if no symptoms occur, you will be returned to the lying position, whereupon a drug that increases your heart rate will be started. Once the heart rate your doctor seeks is reached, you will be raised to the 80° position again for another 20 minutes. When the procedure is completed, if an IV has been inserted, it will then be removed. The test results will be either positive or negative. In the case of a positive test, your

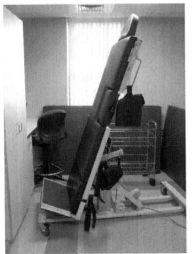

The tilt table procedure involves being strapped to the table to protect you from injury if you pass out. Baseline vital signs are taken, and the table is raised to approximately 80 degrees, where vital signs are monitored, while searching for a dramatic drop in blood pressure, or heart rate.

Figure 6

14

doctor will probably prescribe a beta-blocker. This is a medicine that helps control overreaction of the nerve receptors. If the tilt table is negative, your doctor will look for other reasons causing your symptoms.

If your physician suspects you have an SVT (supraventricular tachycardia) and it has not been documented, there are three ways to document these arrhythmias: The first is called a Holter monitor. A Holter monitor is a recording device that uses 3-7 EKG electrodes connected to the recorder. This monitor is usually used when someone has a frequently occurring arrhythmia. The Holter monitor is good for use from one to seven days, during which time you keep a symptoms log. At the time you have symptoms, you press a button on the Holter monitor, and it marks the spot on the recorder where your symptoms occurred. (*Figure* 7)

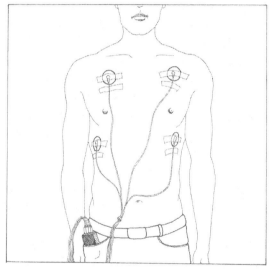

The Holter monitor (on the patient's hip) is a recording device connected via 3-7 electrodes, and is used to monitor patients with frequent arrhythmias.

Figure 7

The second option is called the King of Hearts monitor. This monitor is used for patients who do not have daily symptoms. The King of Hearts monitor is usually worn for 30 days. It works in the same manner as the Holter monitor, for you keep a log of events and push a button to mark the symptomatic events. (*Figure 8*)

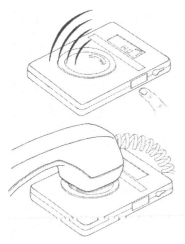

The King of Hearts monitor functions like a Holter Monitor, but it is used for patients with less frequent arrhythmias. It is used to monitor patients for up to thirty days, and the information gathered can be transmitted to the doctor's office by telephone.

Figure 8

The third option is an implantable loop recorder. This device is used with people who experience symptoms rarely but where symptoms are very noticeable when they do occur. The implantable loop recorder can be used from one day to two years. Unlike the Holter monitor and the King of Hearts monitor, which are worn on the outside of the body, the implantable loop recorder requires a minor surgery for insertion within the body. (See, *Figure 9* below)

The placement of the loop recorder may be done in a physician's office or a procedure room at the local hospital. The procedure is performed using a sterile technique (a very clean procedure) where the staff will wear hats and masks.

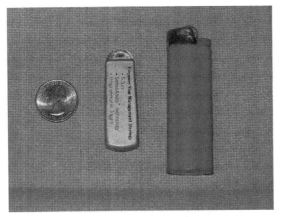

The loop recorder is a small device that requires a small incision for placement, and records long-term information, using a remote to trigger recordings for your doctor's review.

Figure 9

16

The preparation includes washing the area of insertion with a sterile solution and draping it with sterile materials. The sterile materials are bought pre-packaged and are used to reduce the risk of infection. The site of implant is about two inches below the collarbone on the left side of the chest. This area is used because it is closest to the heart. Once the area is prepped and draped, the doctor will use a sterile washing technique and have the assistant put on a sterile gown and gloves on him/her. When the physician is satisfied that the procedure can be done with very little risk of infection, he/she will start by using a numbing agent like a dentist uses novacaine before replacing a filling. Once the area is numb, the doctor will make a 1-2 inch incision, or cut, into the skin. After any bleeding is under control, the physician will use one or two fingers to make a pocket, an area the size of the loop recorder. This is accomplished by separating the skin from the muscle. When the pocket is completed, the doctor will turn to the sterile loop recorder located on the sterile procedure table. He will lift and place the sterile loop recorder in the preformed pocket and suture (sew) the pocket closed. Afterward, a sterile dressing or a Band-Aid will be placed over the surgical site. Once the dressing is applied and the sterile drapes are removed, the representative from the manufacturer of the loop recorder will give you the remote control for the loop recorder and explain how it is used. Whenever you experience symptoms, you will use the remote to record whatever is happening during that time. Then you will contact your doctor, and using the monitor company's programmer, you and your physician can view what occurred during the episodes.

As mentioned earlier, an SVT is supraventricular tachycardia. Supra means above, ventricular means lower chambers of the heart, and tachycardia means going fast. As a general rule, SVTs are not deadly but can cause you to be uncomfortable. The reason they are safer is that the AV node is like a gatekeeper. The faster the signals are sent from the atrium to the AV node, the less these signals are allowed to pass to the ventricles. The SVT can be atrial fibrillation, atrial flutter, atrial tachycardia, AV nodal reentrant tachycardia, or an accessory bypass tract. Each of these are explained in the following paragraphs.

Atrial fibrillation is probably the most familiar, because President George Bush experienced atrial fibrillation during his presidency and the media informed, as well as misinformed, us about its characteristics. The fibrillation part of the arrhythmia means the upper chamber of the heart is beating more than 350 beats per minute in an erratic manner. While atrial fibrillation is the most common or most well known, atrial arrhythmia research articles state that atrial fibrillation affects between 4% and 6% of Americans. There are three types of atrial fibrillation: paroxysmal, persistent, and permanent. Each of these types is treated in a different manner and will be discussed in detail later, while the description is provided as follows.

The Heart Rhythm Society defines paroxysmal atrial fibrillation as an atrial fibrillation that occurs anywhere from seconds to days, and terminates on its own. Persistent atrial fibrillation requires either medication or electrocardioversion to return the heart to normal rhythm; and permanent, or chronic, atrial fibrillation is atrial fibrillation that cannot be terminated with medication or electrocardioversion.

Compared to atrial fibrillation, atrial flutter is a more organized SVT. Atrial flutter is referred to as a macro-reentrant tachycardia, or a big loop. This means the electrical signal travels around the atrium in a clockwise or counter clockwise direction. The majority of these use the isthmus, or the floor of the atrium, which in a normal heart has no electrical conductivity or cannot provide a pathway.

AVNRT, or atrioventricular nodal reentrant tachycardia, is the most common SVT seen in the electrophysiology lab. It is referred to as a micro-reentrant circuit, which means that when the heart developed, it developed two AV nodes, or junction boxes, with the second one coming into action when the main AV node cannot accept an electrical signal, referred to as in refractory. (*See, Drawings A, B, and C*)

The light arrows represent normal electrical conduction while the dark areas represent arrhythmias.

<u>A</u>

A macro-reentrant (large loop) circuit can occur in any chamber of the heart as well as between two chambers and travel in any direction.

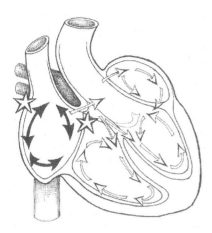

Figure A

<u>B</u>

A micro-reentrant (small loop) circuit is usually only found in AV nodal reentry where the heart can have two AV nodes or junction boxes.

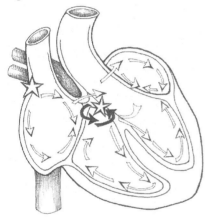

Figure B

<u>C</u>

Focal arrhythmias can initiate from one or many sites in a heart chamber entering the normal electrical system causing higher heart rates. (The drawings depict three focal sites.)

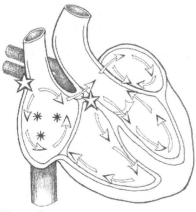

Figure C

19

Atrial tachycardia is not erratic, nor is it a micro or macro-reentrant tachycardia. Atrial tachycardia initiates from a focus other than the sinoatrial node, but the electrical signal goes to the SA node and triggers a tachycardia at different rates, depending on where it strikes the SA node. This arrhythmia is one of the most interesting because it can come from one or more initiation sites but, with newer technologies, may be cured in a timely manner.

The final supraventricular tachycardia is an accessory bypass tract. While the other SVTs use the AV node (the junction box), accessory bypass tracts may or may not use the AV node. Because of the accessory bypass tract, tachycardias can reach much higher heart rates than other SVTs and are a cause for concern. Remembering an earlier discussion, when the heart develops, a skeleton is formed that separates the upper chambers from the lower chambers and separates the upper and lower chambers from each other. With an accessory bypass tract, conductive fibers are present around the mitral and tricuspid valves allowing electrical signals to return to the atria, starting a tachycardia. Depending on the direction the circuit travels, the tachycardia can be easily diagnosed using a 12-lead EKG. This type of bypass tract is referred to as Wolff-Parkinson-White syndrome. If the circuit goes the opposite direction and cannot be easily identified by EKG, it is called a concealed bypass tract.

Turning from the SVTs, let us examine arrhythmias that occur in the ventricles or lower chambers of the heart, PVCs (premature ventricular contractions), ventricular tachycardia, and ventricular fibrillation. PVCs come from ectopic sites outside of the normal electrical system. They may come alone, in twos, or in short runs of more. Some patients describe PVCs as hard heartbeats that get your attention and that happen infrequently. If you think you are having PVCs, you can feel your pulse and notice a rhythm. The heartbeats will be regular and then a beat occurs earlier, followed by a pause, and, finally, a return to a rhythmic pattern.

Not everyone will have PVCs, but age and caffeine intake seem related for those who do have them. Age is a factor we cannot change, and it seems reasonable that the older a person becomes, the more PVCs they may have without major concern. With the medical advancements made, people are living longer than ever before, which, with time, exposes more medical situations not experienced before.

Unlike age, caffeine intake is a factor we can control. A businessman or businesswoman who cannot get out of bed without a cup of coffee, and then continues to have another 10-12 cups during the day, may have more frequent PVCs than a person who has only one or two cups a day. The bottom line is that if you have PVCs, regulate your caffeine intake and you will notice a change in the frequency of PVCs.

When PVCs occur in groups, it is called ventricular tachycardia. Groups of three are referred to as triplets, and more than three are classified as non-sustained or sustained tachycardia. Sustained tachycardia is 15 PVCs in one definition or longer than 15 seconds of PVCs in another definition. Anything less is non-sustained ventricular tachycardia. Ventricular tachycardia can occur at a rate just above 100 beats per minute and rise up to 240 beats per minute. The lower heart rates are, generally, caused by the effects of drugs. This means a cardiologist is aware you have a ventricular tachycardia and prescribes medications to control it.

Along with variable rates, ventricular tachycardia is classified as stable or unstable. Stable ventricular tachycardia is a rhythm that the patient does not know they have, or they might know they have it, but show no symptoms. Some patients are sensitive to changes in their heart rhythm and can tell a healthcare provider when their rhythm changes even though there are no symptoms. Others may happen to be on a heart monitor when the ventricular tachycardia occurs, and it is observed and documented by a medical staff member. Once a member of the staff recognizes ventricular tachycardia, he/she will question the patient about the symptoms.

Unlike stable ventricular tachycardia, patients with unstable ventricular tachycardia are symptomatic. Symptoms may include dizziness, palpitations, blurred vision, and syncope. If a person survives an episode of unstable ventricular tachycardia, there will be a multitude of tests performed to determine the cause of this event. Some of these tests may include stress testing, echocardiography, heart catheterization, and electrophysiologic evaluations. These tests will be explained in another chapter.

Yet another classification of ventricular tachycardia is as monomorphic or polymorphic. A monomorphic tachycardia means that each beat comes from the same site, so when it is represented or viewed on an EKG, each beat looks the same as the previous beat. On the other hand, polymorphic VT, or ventricular tachycardia, means it comes from multiple sites. While two beats in a row may look the same, the third, fourth, and fifth may look different. This is what tells you it comes from multiple sites.

NOTES

CHAPTER 4
Your Doctor Recommends
An Electrophysiology Study

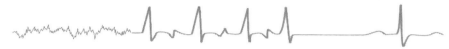

After meeting with your electrophysiologist, an electrophysiology (EP) study has been recommended. The doctor explains that this study will allow for a more accurate treatment of your condition. At this point, a rush of questions and maybe a little uneasiness enter your mind. If you choose to proceed with the EP, it is important that you get all your questions answered and understand the mechanics of the procedure completely. Once the decision has been made to proceed, an appointment will be scheduled for your study. If you are like me, as soon as the doctor walks out of the room or when you return home, more questions will come to mind. Again, it is important to have all your questions answered, so write them down and call the doctor's nurse or assistant to have them answered.

The EP study is an invasive procedure, meaning that the doctor will put catheters into your body to perform the test. Anytime this occurs, it is important to avoid infection, whether you are having blood drawn or having open-heart surgery. You should be aware of these precautions in the preoperative unit or from the hospital staff in your room, throughout your procedure, and until you leave the hospital.

On the day of your procedure, your journey begins in the admitting department. Here, the clerk will enter you into the hospital system. The doctor's office may have given you a packet of information to bring with you, and if not, it could have been faxed or brought by courier to the hospital admitting or outpatient department. You will also need your insurance card. Most hospitals use some form of outpatient unit to prepare you for your EP study. These units help keep your costs and your insurance company's costs down while giving the hospital a chance to discharge patients from the floors, and to have an open room available, should it be needed. Once the admitting clerk has registered you into the hospital system, someone from the hospital transport department or a representative from the outpatient department will escort you to a room in the outpatient department. Here a nurse's aide will weigh you and check your height and then will help you settle into your room. You will change out of your street clothes and into a hospital gown. A good suggestion here would be to ask for a second gown in case you have to leave your room for any reason; you can wear the second gown backwards, and it will keep your backside covered. Before you get into bed, you may want to give a family member anything valuable that you brought with you to the hospital. If you wear glasses, you will want to keep these with you until your procedure. At most of the hospitals where I have worked, you are allowed to take your glasses to the procedure, if you wish. There may be a time when a member of the staff needs to remove your glasses, so help the staff to remember to return them to you at the end of the procedure. If a family member is not available to take your valuables, an aide in the outpatient unit can call the hospital security office for someone who will bring a locking bag to you, and who will give you a receipt for your valuables. At discharge time, you will use that receipt to redeem your valuables.

Now that you are in bed, the nurse's aide will take your vital signs, including heart rate, blood pressure, and oxygen saturation. Next, the nurse will come to your room to complete the unit admission form, including asking about allergies and any concerns you or your family have about the procedure. The doctor's preoperative orders will be reviewed with you, and blood will be drawn for any tests requested. This will be followed by a trip to the x-ray department, if ordered by the doctor, or if it was not completed prior to your coming to the preoperative unit. The next step is to sign a consent form for the procedure. This is a required legal document that allows the hospital to confirm what procedure you are scheduled for and assures the hospital that you understand what will be done during the procedure.

One of the final steps in preparing you for your procedure is shaving the hair in your groin area. Both the left and right groins will be prepped, as the groin is the preferred entry site since the veins and arteries are larger there than in the arms or in the neck. The remaining step comes when the procedure room calls the outpatient unit to alert them that the procedure staff is ready for you. At this point, the nurse or nurse's aide will give you a last opportunity to use the restroom.

Now the hard part is waiting for your turn in the procedure lab. Here is it important for you to know and understand that if you are not the first case of the day, the time you will go for your procedure is just an estimate. When the doctor's office knows you are a "to-follow" or a "next case," they will schedule you to arrive later in the morning. If you are already a patient in the hospital, the consent will be signed in your room and you will wait there.

NOTES

CHAPTER 5
The Electrophysiology Study

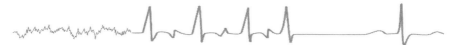

In this chapter, I will explain to you why your electrophysiologist recommended the study for you and what to expect when you enter the procedure room.

First, let me describe an EP study. An electrophysiology study is a procedure to recreate the symptoms you are experiencing, but in a controlled situation. The staff, which is comprised of your doctor and a combination of cardiovascular technologists, x-ray technologists, respiratory therapy technologists, and nurses will use electrode catheters in various areas of your heart to compare your electrical signals to what are considered normal electrical signal values. Then pacing protocols will be used to recreate your symptoms or document your arrhythmia.

There are many ways you may have qualified for an EP study. Strict regulations were adopted in the United States and worldwide medical communities who need EP studies. Some of these include information from a Holter or King of Hearts monitor, information from an implantable loop recorder, unexplained syncope, or something documented during a visit to your physician or in an emergency room. Once you meet any of these criteria, you will be scheduled for the EP study, if you are in agreement that this is reasonable. If you are an outpatient, not already registered in the hospital, you will be directed to admitting first, and then the outpatient unit, where all the preoperative orders will be completed. If you are already a patient in the hospital, these orders will be carried out in your room.

Once your doctor and the electrophysiology staff are ready to perform your procedure, a representative from the lab will contact your unit or floor for "pre-op." This is your chance to use the restroom right before you go into the procedure room or laboratory. The procedure may take from one to eight hours, depending on what is found during the EP study. If a radio-frequency ablation, pacemaker, or implantable cardiac defibrillator is indicated, your time in the lab will be longer than if a negative result occurs, in other words no arrhythmias noted. The above-mentioned procedures will be discussed in later chapters.

In my experience, a typical EP study will take from one to two hours; however, depending upon the findings, the procedure time can be longer. This is why I mentioned earlier that if you are not the first case scheduled in the procedure room, your scheduled time is only an estimate. Please be patient, as your doctor and staff work diligently to ensure that each patient receives the proper intervention needed to achieve the result you and your doctor desire.

When it is time for your procedure, a member of the staff from the lab or hospital transport department will arrive at your room and take you to the lab, either by stretcher or wheelchair. As you enter the room, you will see a lot of equipment. You will notice that the room is chilly. The temperature in these rooms is kept lower to keep the millions of dollars worth of equipment from overheating. To compensate for the lower temperatures, a lab staff member usually has access to a warm blanket, so do not be shy about asking for one.

Let us take a moment and examine the equipment you will see. There are usually three stations used in an EP study: a recording station, a circulator station, and the procedure station. Each station has different equipment that when used all together allows the doctor and staff to complete your procedure in the safest and most efficient manner. At this point, let me explain the equipment you see in the room pictures provided.

At the recording station, (*Figure 10*), you will see screens for the recording system. One of these screens is used to view live electrical signals, and the other is a review

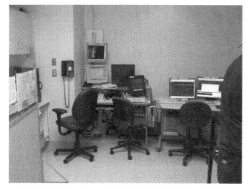

The recording station (desk to right) has live and review monitors where the doctor monitors the electrical signals from your heart as well as the ablation generator, if needed. The desk to the left houses monitors and controls for the x-ray equipment and the stimulator for pacing your heart when needed.

Figure 10

screen, where the recording person can freeze images from the live screen for the doctor to review. Another piece of equipment at the recording station is the stimulator. When connected to the catheters the doctor places in your heart, the stimulator will allow for pacing at rates higher than your normal heart rate. The stimulator is a vital piece of equipment, which uses a wide range of heart rates to narrow down the specific electrical timing that initiates your arrhythmia. A third screen allows the recorder to view x-ray images of the catheter placements.

Another piece of equipment is the ablation generator. I will discuss the use of an ablation generator at a later point.

The circulator is your contact person during the procedure. This staff member is responsible for monitoring your vital signs: heart rate, oxygen saturation, and blood pressure, administering medications, scratching your nose (if requested), and implementing rescue therapies if needed. This station (*Figure 11*) has access to the live screen via a "slave" monitor, a drug-dispensing machine, and two defibrillators.

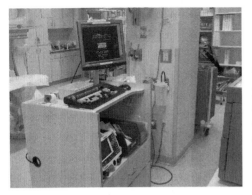

This is the circulator station where your vital signs are monitored and the circulator has access to relaxation medications, supplemental oxygen and the defibrillator, if needed.

Figure 11

The first defibrillator is usually connected to your chest and back by patches before the procedure, and the second is equipped with paddles in case the patches are unsuccessful. Also located at this station is an oxygen meter where extra oxygen is administered according to your level of consciousness.

The procedure station (*Figure 12*) has a hard, flat, narrow table with a thin mattress, an x-ray unit commonly called a C-arm for its shape, catheter connector modules, and a 12-lead EKG cable. Also situated at this station is a blood pressure cuff and pulse oximeter, which measures your heart rate and oxygen saturation. In addition, a separate table with all the equipment needed for the procedure will be on either side of the procedure table.

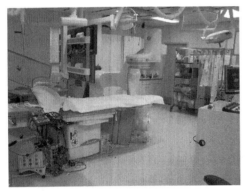

As you entered the procedure room, you noticed the patient table. At the head of the table is the x-ray equipment, while the monitors the doctor will view are at the end of the table and will be positioned once you are on the table.

Figure 12

As you view these three stations, a staff member will help you onto the procedure table from your stretcher or wheelchair. Once you are positioned on the table, the staff will prepare you for the procedure. He/she will give you arm boards, which allow you to keep your arms comfortably at your sides. At this point, the staff member may or may not put soft bracelets on your wrists. These are tied to the table and help refrain you from putting your hands into the sterile work area. Before tying these to the table, the rescue patches will be applied—one to the front of you and the other to your back. Next, one of the staff members will hook up the 12-lead EKG using smaller patches. After all of the wires are attached, a staff member will expose your groin area and place a towel over your genitalia, while leaving access for sheath placement. These areas will be washed with an antiseptic solution to prevent an infection. In addition, the circulator will place oxygen tubing in your nose to regulate supplemental oxygen to your level of consciousness throughout the procedure.

After the above preparation is complete, a staff member will inform the doctor you are ready for the procedure. At this point, the doctor will enter the procedure room to identify you as the patient and confirm with the staff what procedure is being performed. This is also your last chance to have any questions answered before the procedure begins. During this time, the scrub, (doctor's assistant) will put protective lead apron on, as well as a hat and mask, before performing a sterile scrub and entering the room. Here, the scrub will don a sterile gown and gloves and then place a sterile drape over you, leaving the previously cleaned areas exposed for sheath place-ment. The circulator will then administer relaxing medications ordered by your doctor, and the doctor will be completing the sterile scrub. Follow-ing the sterile scrub, your doctor will put on a sterile gown and gloves and enter the room.

Once all the sterile preparation is completed and you are comfortably sedated, the doctor will begin by numbing the groin areas with an agent comparable to novacaine used in a dentist's office. After giving the numb-ing agent ample time to work, the doctor will place sheaths in your groin. A sheath is like an IV, only larger being from 1-4 mm in diameter. It has a one-way valve so a variety of catheters can be placed through it with minimal or no blood loss. The number of sheaths (one to four) depends on which arrhythmia the doctor is trying to identify. The sheaths are put in place by inserting a needle into the vein, and a guide wire through the needle. The needle is then removed and the sheath is placed over the wire. With the wire removed and the sheaths in place, electrode catheters are guided into position in the heart. In a typical three-catheter study, one catheter will be placed in the high right atrium to record signals from the upper chamber of the heart; a second catheter is placed across the His (pronounced, "hiss") bundle (the junction box), to record signals from the low right atrium, through the His bundle, to the upper right ventricle; and a third catheter is placed in the right ventricular apex (the lower chamber). When proper catheter placement has been confirmed, a gathering of information can begin.

The doctor will move from your bedside to the recording station. Your basic electrical measurements will be taken and compared to normal values. If any of these values are out of normal range, they provide one piece of information for a diagnosis. Once the basic measurements are complete, the doctor will begin programmed stimulation. It is important for you to understand that your arrhythmia is initiated by a certain glitch in your electrical system, and the stimulation protocol is used to find the exact timing of this glitch. A generally accepted protocol uses an eight-beat pacing train at 100, 120, and 150 beats per minute and adding one, two, or three early beats. These are used in both the upper and lower chambers of the heart. If the arrhythmia the doctor is trying to recreate is from the lower chamber and pacing from the tip of the lower chamber is negative, the catheter will be moved to a second position. If pacing from both of these sites produces no results, the chance of having a ventricular arrhythmia after you leave the lab is very low. On the other hand, if the doctor is trying to reproduce an atrial arrhythmia and the pacing protocol did not initiate one, the doctor may have the circulator start an IV medication to increase your heart rate. Once your heart rate reaches the goal determined by the doctor, the protocol will be repeated. Again, if the result is negative, there is a very low chance of an atrial arrhythmia occurring after leaving the lab.

It should be duly noted that the description I have given for an electrophysiology study could be modified if there is some documentation that the arrhythmia is present. A limited study may be performed if a cardiac arrest brought you to the hospital. In this situation, the doctor may do only a ventricular pacing protocol to see if ventricular tachycardia can be induced, and if it can, does it deteriorate to ventricular fibrillation? This information can be used when programming an implantable cardiac defibrillator, as discussed in a later chapter.

Now, what if your study was positive? In the event that an atrial arrhythmia was induced, the doctor may opt to use radiofrequency ablation as a curative procedure. This will depend upon the arrhythmia and the capability of the lab to perform such a procedure. In some cases, the atrial arrhythmia will be one that is seen infrequently, and may have a greater chance of success in a university lab where they see that particular rhythm almost daily. Your doctor wants to give you the greatest opportunity for success and in certain situations may suggest this option. Most atrial arrhythmias, however, may be cured by your doctor in the same setting as your EP study.

If your EP study was negative, the catheters will be removed, as well as the sterile drapes, and then a scrub person will remove the sheaths and apply pressure until any bleeding ceases. Finally, you will be returned to your room where you will lie in bed for the doctor-prescribed recovery period. Once this period is complete, you will be discharged to return home or to your hospital room.

If a radiofrequency ablation is recommended to cure your arrhythmia, a fourth sheath may be inserted to allow access of a coronary sinus catheter. This catheter enters the coronary sinus, which is the return pathway of blood from the heart to get more oxygen. A special ablation catheter will need to be used. These catheters are usually larger than those used during the diagnostic test; therefore, one of the sheaths may be exchanged for a larger sheath. Catheter-induced ablation, as described in *Dorland's Medical Dictionary*, is delivery of destructive electrical energy, usually high energy or radiofrequency alternating current, via electrodes on a catheter. In simple terms, ablation blocks the abnormal electrical pathway and redirects the signal down the normal pathway, or eliminates an impulse coming from a single site.

The majority of arrhythmias fall into three categories: macro-reentrant tachycardia, micro-reentrant tachycardia, and focal tachycardia. A macro-reentrant tachycardia is a large-loop tachycardia, whereas a micro-reentrant tachycardia is a small-loop tachycardia. In contrast, a focal tachycardia starts from a single point outside the normal electrical system, but as it progresses, it jumps into the normal system, causing it to go much faster than normal.

If you ask any electrophysiologist which form of ablation is preferred, the answer will be radiofrequency ablation. Radiofrequency was preceded by DC (direct current) ablation, which was found to have some unacceptable outcomes. With the development of radiofrequency ablation, a safe and effective form of ablation has allowed thousands of patients to lead normal lives after their arrhythmias were completely eliminated. While radiofrequency is the standard for ablation, other forms are proving successful, such as cryogenic (freezing), ultrasound, microwave, and alcohol. Each of these forms of ablation seems to have a specific application at this moment, but may replace radiofrequency in the future.

In the following pages, I will describe each of the most prominent arrhythmias that lend themselves to ablation and how your doctor identifies your arrhythmia. These arrhythmias include AVNRT (atrioventricular nodal reentrant tachycardia); AFL (atrial flutter); AT (atrial tachycardia); concealed bypass tract, or WPW (Wolff-Parkinson-White syndrome); A-fib (atrial fibrillation); PVCs (premature ventricular complexes); and right ventricular outflow tachycardia.

NOTES

CHAPTER 6
AVNRT (Atrioventricular Nodal Reentrant Tachycardia)

AVNRT is the most common ablation performed. It is a micro-reentrant circuit, meaning it is a small-loop tachycardia. It also means you have two AV nodes, or junction boxes. Both have been present since birth, but the normal one has been hiding the abnormal one. Something has happened over the years to allow the abnormal site to be activated. (*Figure 13*)

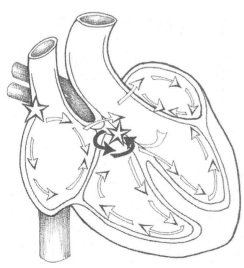

AVNRT starts when the normal AV node will not accept impulses, and the extra AV node (slow pathway) will. Electrical signals are sent to the atrium and ventricle due to the micro-reentrant circuit that causes much higher heart rates than normal. The slow pathway is usually ablated without complications with a complete cure to the arrhythmia.

Figure 13

Your doctor found this arrhythmia during programmed stimulation in the atrium. In the normal heart, the faster the atrium is paced, the longer the delay in the AV node before the electrical signal is passed through to the ventricle. This delay is called the A-H interval, and each time the premature beat is decremented faster, the longer the A-H interval should be until the signal is finally blocked, or not sent to the ventricles. If there is an A-H jump (an increase in the A-H interval more than normal), and the tachycardia starts, this is considered dual AV nodal physiology. The way your doctor eliminates the tachycardia is with ablation of the abnormal pathway. Great care is taken while performing ablation of this abnormal pathway not to ablate the normal pathway, which would require placement of a pacemaker.

Once the doctor finishes ablating the designated site, the atrial protocol is performed again. If no A-H jumps are noted and the tachycardia does not start, the procedure is a success. In some cases the doctor may administer an IV medication to increase your heart rate to simulate an exercise state. If the atrial protocol is run again and the arrhythmia does not occur, this confirms that the arrhythmia has been eliminated.

At the end of this procedure, the sterile drapes will be removed, sheaths will be removed, and pressure will be applied until all bleeding is under control, and you will be returned to your room for the doctor-designated recovery period.

NOTES

CHAPTER 7
AFL (Atrial Flutter)

Atrial flutter is a macro-reentrant (large-loop) tachycardia. In the normal heart, when the electrical signal is initiated, it spreads out over the whole right atrium and converges at the AV node, where it is allowed to pass through to the ventricles. There are no electrical signals that pass along the floor, or the bottom, of the atrium, as this is part of the skeleton of the heart. With atrial flutter, some electrical fibers are in the floor in the atrium, allowing the signal to make a full circle in the atrium. Because the AV node is not involved in this circuit, the atrial heart rate can get quite fast. As the signals enter the AV node, not all of them are allowed to pass to the ventricles. The faster the signals reach the AV node, the fewer of these signals conduct to the ventricles. You may hear your atrial flutter as 2:1, 3:1 or 4:1 atrial flutter, which means that for each two, three, or four atrial beats that reach the AV node, one is allowed to pass to the ventricles.

You may enter the lab already in atrial flutter, or your doctor may induce it during the diagnostic study. Once you are in atrial flutter, your doctor can determine whether you have clockwise or counterclockwise flutter. This is determined by using electrograms from the catheters already in place, seeing which atrial signal is first, and which is last. The majority of atrial flutters are isthmus dependent. The isthmus is the floor of the atrium, and while there are other types of atrial flutter, they are so few and far between that I will only describe isthmus-dependent flutter.

Once your doctor has determined that your arrhythmia is atrial flutter, an ablation catheter will be inserted. The doctor may use a large-tip catheter, as the isthmus is a large area to ablate compared to the small areas ablated in other arrhythmias. If you refer to the illustration (*Figure 14*), you can see the amount of tissue area that needs to be electrically isolated using long high-energy lesions. An important side note is that this area is not supposed to conduct electrical impulses in a normal conduction system, and ablating is relatively safe.

After your doctor feels enough ablation has been completed, pacing from both sides of the atrium will be performed. If the signal still crosses the isthmus, more ablation will be done. When pacing from both sides is completed with no signal crossing the isthmus, the procedure is considered successful, and sterile drapes will be removed, sheaths will be removed, pressure will be held until all bleeding has stopped, and you will be returned to your room for the doctor-prescribed recovery period.

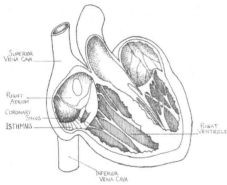

SUPERIOR
VENA CAVA

RIGHT
ATRIUM

CORONARY
SINUS

ISTHMUS

RIGHT
VENTRICLE

INFERIOR
VENA CAVA

The isthmus is the area between the coronary sinus and tricuspid valve to the inferior vena cava. In a normal heart, no electrical impulses travel across this area. With typical atrial flutter, the isthmus completes the macro reentrant circuit. Once this area is ablated, the electrical impulses do not conduct across this area and the arrhythmia is cured.

Figure 14

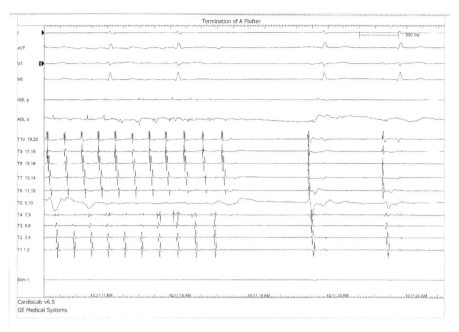

Figure 15

On the left side of the above electrogram, the large deflections in the first four lines represent the ventricles with very little activity seen between each deflection. The lower ten lines represent atrial activity from a catheter in the right atrium. Notice there are as many as four atrial beats for each ventricular beat. The diagnosis here is atrial flutter. The right side of the electrogram shows only one atrial beat for each ventricular beat, indicating successful ablation of the flutter circuit, and return to normal rhythm.

NOTES

CHAPTER 8
AT (Atrial Tachycardia)

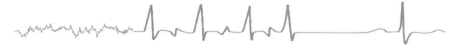

Atrial tachycardia is a focal arrhythmia, meaning that it originates from a single site, and while this occurs from a single site, there may be many sites requiring ablation. Your doctor identified you as having atrial tachycardia while performing atrial-pacing protocols. When the rhythm is initiated, the earliest atrial signal comes in the high right atrium catheter. (*Figure 16*)

I have seen two methods of ablating atrial tachycardia: "leapfrogging" catheters or using one of the mapping systems available to electrophysiology labs. Leapfrogging catheters involve keeping your tachycardia going while moving a second catheter around the suspected area for an earlier atrial signal than the one in the first catheter. When an earlier signal is found, then the first catheter is moved looking for an even earlier signal. This is continued until no earlier signal can be found. At this point, energy will be applied until the tachycardia stops. The problem with leapfrogging is when there is more than one site that causes the arrhythmia. An example would be that your doctor is looking for the earliest signal in one area, when the rate and look of the tachycardia change. This means that there is a second site, and the doctor will have to move the catheters to the new site looking for the earliest signal. After the doctor moves the catheters to the new site, the rate and look of the previous tachycardia recur, and the doctor needs to move the catheters back to the first site he was mapping. If these sites keep changing, they will produce a long procedure. With the advent of mapping systems, leapfrogging catheters, while still used in some labs, has diminished greatly for atrial tachycardia ablation.

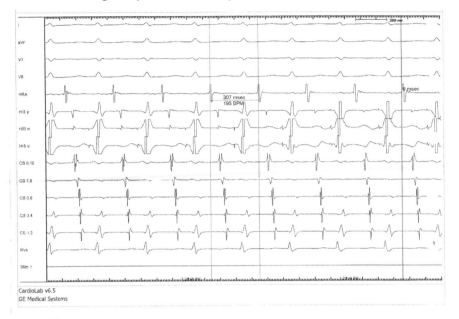

Figure 16

In the above electrogram, you can see the earliest electrical signal is just after the vertical line in the HRA channel, with those in the HIS and CS channels coming later. With the HRA signal first, and the heart rate of 195 beats per minute, a diagnosis of atrial tachycardia is confirmed.

A mapping system allows the doctor to create a 3D image of the heart chamber of interest. Once this is accomplished, the arrhythmia is started and recorded. Each beat is mapped to its point of origin. If all of them map to the same point, this is when the doctor will ablate. One of the mapping systems allows the doctor to record the rhythm and map the beats recorded, even if the rhythm stops. With leapfrogging and other mapping systems, you have to be in the tachycardia to find the site for ablation. This means that if your tachycardia stops, it needs to be started again before the ablation site can be mapped, which, in turn, adds more time to the procedure. Yet another advantage of the mapping system is with multiple sites. If the doctor is working on one site and another tachycardia starts, it can be recorded and dealt with after the first site is ablated. This has greatly helped in reducing the procedure time.

Once the doctor has ablated the site or sites, the atrial protocol will be run again. If the arrhythmia cannot be induced, a drug may be given to increase your heart rate, whereupon, if the arrhythmia still cannot be started, this will be the endpoint of your procedure. Again, the catheters and sheaths will be removed and pressure will be held on the sheath insertion site until all bleeding has stopped, and then you will be transported back to your room for the doctor-prescribed recovery period.

NOTES

CHAPTER 9
Concealed Bypass Tracts and (WPW) Wolff-Parkinson-White Syndrome

Bypass tracts, whether concealed on unconcealed, are macro-reentrant circuits that may not use the AV node. These are located in the electrical circuit on the left or right side of the heart, and allow atrial signals to pass to the ventricles at faster rates than if the AV node was involved. The bypass tract involves the mitral valve, the valve between the left atrium and left ventricle, and is the area your doctor will concentrate on ablating. The difference between a concealed bypass tract and Wolff-Parkinson-White syndrome is the direction the circuit runs. If it runs in one direction, there is evidence of a bypass tract that can be seen on a 12-lead EKG. This is called Wolff-Parkinson-White syndrome. If it runs the other direction, it is called a concealed bypass tract, because it cannot be identified on a 12-lead EKG. To eliminate either of these bypass tracts, your doctor will need to isolate the earliest atrial signal from the left or right side of the heart.

As mentioned previously, the coronary sinus catheter provides information with electrical signals from the left side of the heart. When your arrhythmia is initiated, atrial signals in the coronary sinus catheter are earlier than atrial signals from either the right atrial catheter or the His catheter. Once your doctor has determined that a bypass tract is present, and the arrhythmia can be started and stopped, the next step is deciding how to get the ablation catheter to the site.

The left side of the heart is the high-pressure side, which is responsible for sending oxygenated blood to all parts of the body, including the brain and other vital organs. The left side of the heart can be accessed using the retrograde (against the flow of blood) method, or the transseptal method. The retrograde method involves putting a sheath in the artery of the right groin and maneuvering the catheter through the aorta, over the aortic arch, and prolapsing (bending) the catheter across the aortic valve, and into the left ventricle, which gives your doctor access to the ventricular side of the mitral valve. If access to the atrial side of the mitral valve is your doctor's goal, then the catheter will also need to be prolapsed across this valve.

With the transseptal method, your doctor can access the left side of the heart from the right side. This is accomplished by using a long, curved sheath against the atrium septum (the tissue that separates the right atrium from the left atrium), and then pushing a long, curved needle through the sheath and across the septum. The sheath is guided over the needle, and once the sheath is in place, the needle is removed, and the ablation catheter is in place. If your doctor needs access to the ventricular side of the mitral valve, the catheter may be curled and pushed across the valve.

Both methods of left-sided access are relatively safe, but your doctor may choose one over the other depending on his/her experience and success rate. Some options he/she may take into consideration with the retrograde method are that the coronary arteries that supply blood to the heart originate just above the aortic valve, and could be damaged with a misplaced catheter. Crossing one or two valves also changes the maneuverability of the catheter, and in a taller or larger person, catheter length may become an issue. On the other hand, in using the transseptal method, if the needle slips, a hole may puncture the sac surrounding the heart and blood may seep into the sac. If this occurs, a drain must be placed in the sac until the bleeding stops. While these complications rarely occur, they are events your doctor considers before choosing a left atrial access method.

After achieving access, the catheter has to be directed to the ablation site. This site is determined by atrial signals from the coronary sinus catheter. The five sets of electrode pairs are used as markers to guide your doctor to the ablation site. If the earliest atrial signal is in the second, third, or fourth electrode pair, the arrhythmia is bracketed between the first and fifth electrode pairs. Your doctor uses these markers for ablation catheter placement and energy application. In hearts containing a small coronary sinus, a catheter may not be able to reach the back of the heart, and the earliest atrial signal will be in the first electrode pair. In this case, the ablation catheter is moved along an imaginary line, continuing from the catheter, until the earliest atrial signal is found, and energy is applied to eliminate the bypass tract. When a change in the coronary sinus electrical signals appears, ablation is stopped. If your arrhythmia was Wolff-Parkinson-White, your doctor will verify by the 12-lead EKG, to see if it is registering normal. (Compare the EKGs on next page) (*Figure 17*) In the case of a concealed bypass tract, a normal progression of the atrial signals in the coronary sinus catheter is an indication to stop ablating.

Once ablation is stopped, atrial protocols will be performed again. If the arrhythmia is initiated, more energy will be applied until after the atrial protocol does not initiate the arrhythmia, indicating a successful ablation. At this point, catheters and sheaths will be removed and pressure will be held at the site until all bleeding ceases. Finally, you will be returned to your room for the recovery period.

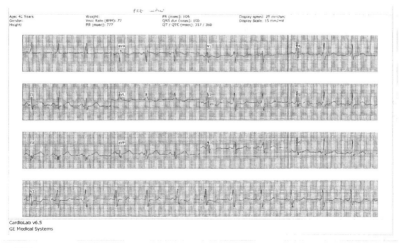

Figure 17A

These EKGs are from the same person. Figure 17A shows, when compared a slurring of the AV interval, which is an indication of Wolff-Parkinson-White syndrome. In this case the doctor found the spot causing the arrhythmia and ablated it. When compared to the above EKG, Figure 17B shows no evidence of slurring (a delta wave), and after additional testing, it was concluded the ablation was successful.

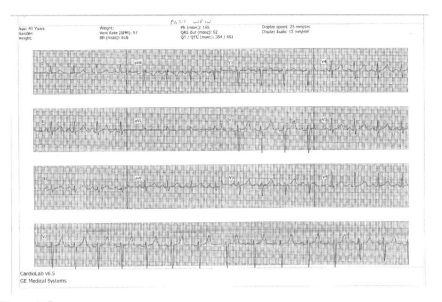

Figure 17B

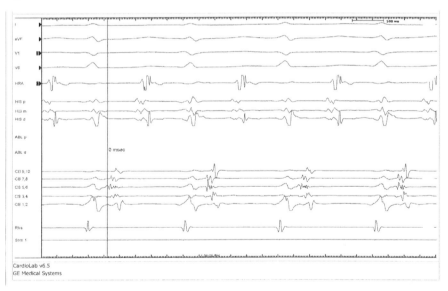

Figure 18

In the above electrogram, one can see the earliest beat after the vertical line is in CS 5, 6. All of the signals from the CS catheter are earlier than those from the HRA or HIS channels, indicating a bypass tract from the left side. (Remember the coronary sinus catheter allows electrical signals from the left side of the heart to be seen without entering the arterial system.) Also, with CS 5, 6 being earlier than any of the other CS channels, the arrhythmia is known as being "bracketed" (surrounded), and the doctor will focus on ablating in that area.

NOTES

CHAPTER 10
AF (Atrial Fibrillation)

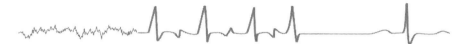

Atrial fibrillation (AF) is an arrhythmia that has befuddled the medical community for years. Some think A-fib is a focal arrhythmia caused by an early atrial beat, while others believe it is initiated from multiple sites in an erratic manner. No matter how it starts, we know atrial fibrillation can cause the atrium to beat up to 600 beats per minute. At these high rates, there is little time for the atrium to fill with blood before it pushes its volume to the ventricles. In a normal heart, the atrium supplies 30% of the total blood distributed with each heartbeat. As a result, when you are in atrial fibrillation, you may observe a lack of energy, or even feel palpitations. These palpitations can occur due to the erratic heart rate, and you may also feel the erratic heartbeat while taking your pulse.

While you are concerned with the physical effects of atrial fibrillation, your doctor is concerned with the results. If the atrium is beating at these high rates, up to 600 beats per minute, the blood in the atrium swirls like water going down a drain in the sink. This lends itself to forming emboli (clots) in the atrium, which can cause a stroke if allowed to reach the brain. When any doctor finds a patient is in atrial fibrillation, one of his/her concerns is putting the patient on blood thinners to avoid the formation of these emboli. The next step is to identify which type of atrial fibrillation is present and how it can be treated.

According to *Braunwald's Heart Disease, A Textbook of Cardiovascular Medicine, Eighth Edition*, after two or more episodes, atrial fibrillation is considered recurrent. If recurrent atrial fibrillation resolves spontaneously, it is designated as paroxysmal. If it occurs beyond seven days, it is termed persistent. Persistent atrial fibrillation also encompasses longstanding atrial fibrillation (generally classified as lasting longer than one year), which usually leads to permanent atrial fibrillation.

When your family practitioner diagnoses you have atrial fibrillation, medical therapy is the first line of treatment. If your doctor is not familiar with the treatment for AF, a cardiologist may be consulted. Once a patient is under the care of a cardiologist, other options become available. The majority of people with paroxysmal atrial fibrillation are successfully treated with medication. However, some patients require the use of additional treatment options, because their AF is not well controlled with medication, only. The options for paroxysmal atrial fibrillation, and persistent atrial fibrillation patients are either surgical or radiofrequency ablation. If your atrial fibrillation allows your heart rate to achieve rates that make you uncomfortable, even with medication, you will want to discuss further options with your cardiologist or electrophysiologist.

The surgical ablation is called the Maze procedure. To accomplish this procedure, you are taken to a surgical suite where you are put under a general anesthetic while your heart is exposed. The surgeon opens the atria, whereupon a checkerboard-shaped pattern is created. The idea is to form many squares in the atria, which will not allow electrical stimulus to pass to the other parts of the heart. The Maze procedure has a higher success rate when compared to radiofrequency ablation. Unfortunately, two of the downfalls of selecting the Maze procedure are a higher risk of infection, and a longer recovery period than radiofrequency ablation.

Radiofrequency ablation for the treatment of atrial fibrillation is a relatively new procedure, when compared to having surgery; nevertheless, it is making great strides in acceptable success rates. There are many considerations when faced with an atrial fibrillation that is difficult to ablate, but two stand out as the gold standard at this time. These are pulmonary vein isolation, and pulmonary vein isolation plus lines of block between the veins.

The pulmonary veins are thought to be responsible for the majority of the abnormal signals that trigger atrial fibrillation. These veins return blood from the lungs to the left atrium, which accounts for about 30% of the normal blood flow with each heartbeat. Atrial fibrillation ablation has become more commonly used with the advancement of mapping system technologies.

After one or two transseptal punctures have been completed and sheaths placed across the septum, which has been previously described, a catheter will be placed into the left atrium to create a virtual image of the chamber and the pulmonary veins. Once the image is complete, a circular catheter with as many as 20 electrodes may be placed around the openings of each vein to measure the electrical signals. If one of these veins has no signals, it can be ignored, and your doctor can concentrate on ablating, or isolating the other three veins. Another way to map the veins is using a soft basket-type catheter in the veins. These catheters have 8 splines (rows) for the eight electrodes on each spline. By placing this catheter in the pulmonary vein, your doctor can see not only the signals around the vein, but he/she can also see how deep in the vein these signals occur. If using this catheter, your doctor can narrow the spot of ablation between 2 of the 64 electrodes. This method may take longer than ablating where the signals exit the vein, and enter the atrium, as well as being more tedious in maneuvering the ablation catheter.

When using a mapping system, each spot of ablation is marked on the virtual image, allowing your doctor to visualize the complete isolation of each vein. When the ablation is complete, the circular catheter can once again be placed at the opening of each vein to confirm no electrical signals remain.

Besides pulmonary vein isolation, alone, your doctor may prefer to also ablate between the veins. When complete, your doctor can see a line of ablation between the inside and outside walls of the atrium as well as the roof and the floor. Upon completion of these lines of ablation, your doctor can manipulate the catheter along these areas to ensure no electrical signals remain.

The best advantage of using the radiofrequency versus surgical ablation is the recovery period. Once your doctor deems the procedure is successful, the catheters and sheaths will be removed and pressure held until all bleeding is stopped. Then you will be returned to your room for a short recovery period before being released from the hospital.

Having discussed medical and ablative procedures for atrial fibrillation, what options are available for those who do not respond to either procedure and continue to be symptomatic? That group can include paroxysmal, persistent, and permanent atrial fibrillation patients, and the favored treatment is an AV node ablation. This procedure involves disconnecting communication between the atrium and the ventricle. It is important to understand that once this procedure is completed, you will be pacemaker dependent. This means, in order to keep your heart rate in a normal range, you will need a pacemaker, which will be discussed in a later chapter. Once a pacemaker has been inserted, you will no longer experience the rapid heart rate and palpitations that made you feel uncomfortable.

NOTES

CHAPTER 11
PVCs (Premature Ventricular Contractions) and RVOT VT (Right Ventricular Outflow Tract Ventricular Tachycardia)

PVCs (premature ventricular contractions) are beats that occur in the ventricle, or lower chamber, from focal points. They are earlier than if conducted in the normal electrical system, and may feel stronger than normal heartbeats, giving you a palpitation. PVCs may occur alone or in groups, and if these groups reach 15 beats, they meet the criteria to be called ventricular tachycardia. As we grow older, the cells in the heart stretch, allowing for abnormal electrical conduction, including premature, or early beats. These beats occur more frequently when stimulated by influences like heavy caffeine use. No matter what causes the PVCs, if they are a bother, you want them to go away. After consulting with your cardiologist, or electrophysiologist, and documenting the PVCs are causing your symptoms, you and your doctor need to consider ablation as a treatment.

If you have chosen to proceed with a PVC ablation, your EP doctor will use "pace mapping," or a mapping system, to identify the site or sites of your PVCs. Both methods require recording your PVCs after all of the catheters are in place. With pace mapping, the PVCs are recorded in a 12-lead EKG format, either printed or stored, in a split review screen format. Using this information, the doctor then determines the PVCs origination area. The doctor will then manipulate the ablation catheter to different locations, pacing through the catheter and comparing the 12-lead EKG pacing with the one from your PVCs. When each lead matches perfectly, energy will be applied. (*Figure 19*) While it may take a few applications of energy, once the ablation is complete, there will be no PVCs present at your resting heart rate, or when ventricular pacing protocols are performed.

If your doctor prefers using a mapping system, the PVCs will be recorded and traced to their origination point. When a few of these beats originate at the same point, the doctor will apply energy until no more PVCs are present. As with pace mapping, when the ablation is complete, there will be no PVCs present at rest or during pacing.

Upon completion of the ablation, the sheaths and catheters will be removed and pressure will be applied until all bleeding stops. You will then be returned to your room for the recovery period.

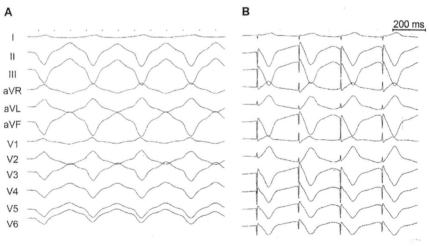

Figure 19

When an arrhythmia starts in a focal area, pace mapping is one strategy to find and ablate it. (A) is a 12-lead EKG of the arrhythmia and (B) pacing in the general vicinity of the arrhythmia. When the pace map looks the same as the arrhythmia in all 12 leads, this is considered a good spot to apply ablation energy.

As mentioned earlier, if there are 15 or more PVCs in a row, it is called ventricular tachycardia. Ventricular tachycardia may be classified as monomorphic or polymorphic, and stable or unstable. Monomorphic ventricular tachycardia is an arrhythmia that originates from one site, meaning every beat looks the same. Polymorphic ventricular tachycardia originates from many sites, and each beat can look different, or some can look the same but others do not. Stable refers to your vital signs—blood pressure, oxygen saturation, heart rate, and level of consciousness—and how your body reacts to any changes while you are in your arrhythmia. If you are unable to respond to hospital staff members, have a dramatic drop in blood pressure, or lose consciousness, this is considered an unstable arrhythmia. An unstable polymorphic ventricular tachycardia lends itself to an implantable cardiac defibrillator for therapy. At the other end of the spectrum, a stable monomorphic ventricular tachycardia lends itself to radiofrequency ablation for therapy. Right ventricular outflow tract ventricular tachycardia is one of these rhythms.

As indicated by its name, right ventricular outflow tract ventricular tachycardia originates from the outflow tract at the right ventricle. Your doctor has identified this by viewing a 12-lead EKG while you were in your arrhythmia. Once the diagnosis is confirmed, your doctor will use either pace mapping, or the mapping system, to locate the exact spot for ablation. Upon completion of the radiofrequency application, your doctor will try to reinitiate the rhythm, and if it cannot be started, the procedure is considered successful. At this point, catheters and sheaths will be removed and pressure applied until all bleeding ceases. You will then be returned to your room for the recovery period, and discharged from the hospital.

NOTES

CHAPTER 12
Pacemakers

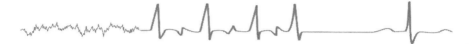

I mentioned in the previous chapter that our heart has three pacemakers. The sinoatrial (SA) node is the main pacemaker of the heart, regulating the heart rate between 60 and 100 beats per minute, and originating in the high right atrium. Once the SA node initiates a heartbeat, the electrical signal spreads throughout the right atrium, into the left atrium, meeting at the atrioventricular (AV)node. It then passes through the AV node to the ventricles, where it spreads over the right and left ventricles, and the heart squeezes oxygenated blood out to the body. If the SA node is diseased, the AV node can provide a heart rate between 40 and 60 beats per minute, and if the AV node fails, the ventricle can provide heart rates between 20 and 40 beats per minute.

As we age, similar to a car, some of our parts start failing. If the SA node does not send signals in a rhythmic pattern to the AV node, it can be termed as having sinus node dysfunction, or sick sinus syndrome. If the sinus node sends signals to the AV node in a rhythmic pattern, but the AV node does not pass these on to the ventricles, it is termed heart block. Both of these electrical problems lend themselves to a pacemaker as therapy. An implantable cardiac pacemaker provides backup to the heart's pacemakers. It does two things—it either senses or paces. For example, let us say your pacemaker is programmed to 60 beats per minute. If your heart beats 60 beats per minute or faster, the pacemaker senses this rate and does nothing but continue to monitor from beat to beat. If your pacemaker does not see a beat of 60 or above, it will send an electrical impulse creating a paced beat. In other words, when you have a pacemaker implanted, your heart rate will not go below your doctor-programmed lowest rate.

There are three types of pacemakers: single-chamber, dual-chamber, and biventricular pacemakers. (*Figure 20*) The remaining part of the system is the leads, which are either active or passive fixation. Active fixation leads have a small helix, or screw, that is screwed into the heart. Passive fixation leads have three or four tines, or little prongs, which are placed in the trabeculae (a network of fibers) of the heart. Both types of leads are recognized as foreign bodies, and over time, the body forms scar tissue around the lead tips, which keeps them in place.

The single-chamber pacing system includes the generator, which can be programmed to pace either the right atrium, or right ventricle, with one pacing lead. A dual-chamber pacing system can be programmed to pace in the right atrium, right ventricle, or both chambers, depending on what your doctor determines is best. A biventricular pacemaker system involves a generator and three leads—one in the right atrium, one in the right ventricle, and one in the left ventricle. The left ventricular lead can be placed through a branch of the coronary sinus that covers the left ventricle, or the lead can be directly attached to the top of the left ventricle, which requires a surgical procedure.

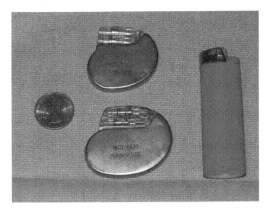

These are two different pacemaker generators. The larger one has more room for a larger battery, and should last longer than the smaller generator.

Figure 20

The biventricular pacemaker is a special system for people with enlarged hearts that have a weakened pumping action, due to the abnormal timing of the electrical system. When these pacemaker systems are placed, your doctor can program the system to mimic a normal timing cycle in the weakened heart, which may reduce the symptoms of the weakened heart. (See, fluoroscopic view of biventricular device below.) (*Figure 21*)

There are some basic parameters included in all pacemakers, such as lower rate—the lowest number of beats per minute your doctor wants your heart to beat; the upper rate—the fastest number of beats per minute your doctor will allow the pacemaker to pace before letting your heart take over; sensitivity—the electrical signals your doctor will let the pacemaker see; and output—the amount of energy used for each pacemaker to beat to ensure contraction of the heart occurs. In dual-chamber and biventricular pacemakers, the AV delay, or the time from when the atrium paces, or beats on its own until the ventricle is paced, and in biventricular pacemakers, the timing interval between when the right ventricle and left ventricles are paced.

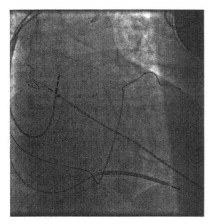

This is a fluoroscopic view of a biventricular device at the finish of the implant. In the upper right, the generator is seen with the three leads emerging. On the left side of the spine (J-shaped) is the atrial lead—over the spine in the middle of the picture is the left ventricular lead (placed through the coronary sinus), and in the lower right, the right ventricular lead can be seen.

Figure 21

While all pacemaker systems have the same basic parameters, the item that separates one company's pacemaker from the others are the extended parameters (bells and whistles) of the device. Some of these are histograms—recorded electrograms, energy-saving algorithms, and sensors, as well as lead impedance trends.

The histograms record what the pacemaker sees and does. They let your doctor know (1) how often your heart beats on its own, versus how often the pacemaker is used; (2) how often the sensor raises the paced heart rate; (3) checks lead impedance trends, which alert your doctor to possible lead failures; and (4) when you have had events that the pacemaker stored as snapshots (recordings of electrical activity outside the normal programmed parameters of the pacemaker).

Stored electrograms provide additional information for your doctor beyond histograms. Using preset limits, your pacemaker will record and store a number of electrograms for events that fall outside the preset values. When you visit your doctor's office, these electrograms can be reviewed and used to adjust your pacemaker to best serve you. These electrograms may also reveal arrhythmias, other than bradycardia, that initially required the placement of the pacemaker system.

Lead impendance trends are another form of information recorded by your pacemaker. Your doctor can use this information to see abrupt changes in lead impedances, which identify possible lead fractures, or leads that may become disconnected from the generator.

Besides collecting information that allows your doctor to fine tune your pacemaker, all pacemaker companies have strived to extend the life of pacemakers. A pacemaker generator contains a small battery, which only achieves an output of 2.5 volts. Compare this generator to a 9-volt battery that is used in many of the children's toys. To get more energy from these batteries, engineers use voltage doublers. When implantable pacemakers were programmed to 3.5 or 5.0 volts output, it only allowed a pacemaker to last for three to five years before needing replacement. Pacemaker companies heard from patients, as well as doctors, that pacemakers needed to last longer. In response to this request, manufacturers have developed energy-saving algorithms. These algorithms test how much energy it takes to produce a contraction at a predetermined interval. Once the energy required is determined, pacemaker output is automatically reset to a value a little higher, allowing a safety margin to ensure a contraction for every pacemaker output. These algorithms have increased pacemaker longevity from two to five years beyond previous pacemakers. Let me add here, it must be noted that longevity depends on the energy required to produce a heart contraction, how often the pacemaker needs to work, and the bells and whistles that have been programmed.

Another "extra" available with pacemakers is a sensor. In the normal heart, as the workload increases, the heart rate increases to supply an adequate blood flow. This means you need a higher heart rate if you are digging a ditch, cooking dinner, or taking a brisk walk. Some people cannot achieve a higher heart rate on their own, and a pacemaker programmed to 60 beats per minute will only pace at 60, even when exercising. If you fall into this category, adding a sensor is the answer. Most pacemakers have a sensor that is a vibratory crystal, meaning that when the crystal vibrates faster than the lower rate, the rate will increase to supply adequate blood flow. While the vibratory crystal is the most common type of sensor, others are now available, or are pending in trials. These include one that uses changes in chest pressure when breathing in and out, and one that uses temperature changes.

Pacemaker and lead technology is changing every day, trying to mimic a normal heart rate for those who need the help. Your doctor is always being updated with information on these changes, to recommend the best pacemaker system for your lifestyle. With this noted, let us turn attention to how these systems are implanted, and what you can expect.

Whether you are already in the hospital, or you enter as an outpatient, the preoperative orders need to be completed before you enter the procedure room. These orders may include a chest x-ray, blood work, initial vital signs, and a consent form for the procedure. Also, your doctor will dictate a history and physical, which gives the staff background information on you and confirms the procedure to be performed. At this time, an intravenous antibiotic will also be started to help prevent any type of infection. Once the preoperative orders are completed, and the procedure room staff are ready to begin, you will be transported by wheelchair or stretcher to the procedure room.

Upon entering the room, you will notice that it is cold. This temperature setting is to keep all of the equipment from overheating, thus allowing your procedure to be accomplished in a safe and efficient manner. Some of this equipment includes the x-ray table with the x-ray equipment at the head of the bed, recording equipment, and normal rescue equipment used in procedure rooms. At this time, the staff will introduce themselves and help you get situated on the x-ray table. You may also request, or a staff member may offer, a warm blanket to offset the cool room temperature. You may also be offered a pillow for under your knees, which eases the pressure on your back. Armboards will be extended, making the table seem wider than its actual size, and EKG leads will be attached to your chest to monitor your heart rate throughout the procedure. A blood pressure cuff and oxygen tubing will be put in place on your arm and in your nose. The supplemental oxygen helps maintain adequate oxygen saturation while relaxing medications are being administered. For most pacemaker implants, these medications keep the patient comfortable, but in certain situations, a general anesthesia may be used. Because the relaxing medications may make you forget where you are, the staff may use soft restraints on your wrists, so you do not accidentally raise your hands into the sterile work area, during the procedure.

Next, the staff will put on hats and masks, if not already done, before opening the sterile equipment for the procedure and applying the sterile prep solution to your skin. If you have hair on the upper half of your chest, it may be shaved, or not, depending on your doctor's choice. Both ways have a similarly low rate of infection. The site prepared can depend on whether you are right or left-handed, as pacemakers are usually placed in the opposite shoulder, due to less daily activity; and whether or not you shoot a shotgun or rifle, again placing it in the opposite shoulder; if there a history of mastectomy, or removal of a breast, again, the opposite side is preferred; or if there is a known venous occlusion, or blocked vein, on the left or right side. You and your doctor should decide on the site to be used, and this should be confirmed with the staff. Once the site is confirmed, the prep solution may be applied. In some instances, both the left and right sides are prepped and left exposed in case the chosen site is unacceptable. Then the opposite site may be quickly accessed, saving the time it would take to prepare the other side.

Once the sterile prep is dry, the scrub tech, or doctor's assistant, performs a sterile scrub and puts on a sterile gown and gloves. The scrub tech will set up the sterile equipment table and place the sterile drapes around the work site. See, (*Figure 22*).

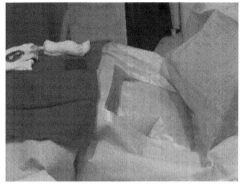

This patient is ready for the doctor to begin the implant. The patient's head is to the right with only a small work area exposed to help reduce the chances of infection.

Figure 22

Do not be surprised if the sterile drapes cover your face. A small area or tent is built from the neck up to avoid moisture from a sneeze or cough contacting the operative site. Other sterile drapes are applied until only the entry site is exposed. From this point forward, the staff member circulating (your contact person) will administer relaxing medications prescribed on the doctor's orders, monitor your vital signs, and scratch your nose if needed. Do not be shy. Speak up if you are uncomfortable. Your doctor and his staff want you to go through this procedure as easily as possible.

Once the sterile preparation is completed and the equipment is ready, the doctor will perform a sterile scrub, and put on a sterile gown and gloves. To begin the procedure, a numbing medicine, like novacaine at the dentist's office, is used to numb the work area. Then a small incision is made to allow access for the leads and a place for the generator to be placed. Here, the doctor will use electrocautery to stop any bleeding, and the tissue is then dissected until the doctor can see the muscle. Next, comes the hardest part of the procedure: the doctor will separate just enough skin from the muscle to form a pacemaker pocket. During pocket formation, you may feel tugging and a little pain, but do not worry, this will only last a few seconds. Once the pocket is formed, your doctor will use a needle and a syringe to access the vein, which is located under the collarbone, which leads to your heart. After access is achieved, the syringe is removed from the needle, and a J-tipped guide wire is placed through the needle, and the needle is removed. This process is repeated if the pacemaker system being implanted requires two or more leads. After gaining access, a peel-away introducer (sheath) is placed over each wire, and the leads are inserted

81

through the introducers. The sheaths are then peeled away, leaving only the pacemaker leads in the vein. Your doctor will then direct the leads to the targeted areas and, if using an active-fixation lead, will deploy the helix, or screw. With the leads in place, measurements are taken, and if they are satisfactory, the leads will be secured in the pacemaker pocket. If they are not satisfactory, the lead will be repositioned and, once satisfactory numbers are achieved, it will be secured in the pacemaker pocket.

While your doctor was placing the leads, a pacemaker company representative or knowledgeable staff member was programming your pacemaker generator to the doctor's specifications. Once the leads are secured and the pacemaker is programmed, the pacemaker is given to the scrub tech, who in turn, gives it to the doctor. The doctor then places the leads in the proper receptacles and secures them using the set screws provided. The doctor may tug on the lead, or leads, to make sure it (they) will not separate from the generator. After the doctor is satisfied that the pacemaker systems is functioning properly, the excess lead, or lead not in the vein, will be coiled, with the pacemaker generator on top, and placed in the pacemaker pocket. Finally, the pacemaker pocket will be closed. This is usually accomplished using one or two layers of dissolvable suture for the tissue, and a layer of dissolvable or non-dissolvable suture to close the skin. If non-dissolvable suture is used, the stitches will need to be removed at the doctor's office in 10-14 days. When the doctor is finished with the procedure, a sterile dressing is applied to the site, followed by removal of the sterile drapes. If the doctor requests any other programming, it may be completed at this point, or when you are returned to your room for recovery. You will then be transported back to your room.

Some doctors like a chest x-ray taken immediately after the procedure, while others prefer to wait until just before you leave the hospital. Either way is acceptable, as this x-ray provides a template to compare with x-rays taken at a later date in case of lead dislodgement or lead fracture is suspected.

When you return to your room, you will again be monitored for heart rate, blood pressure, and oxygen saturation. The head of your bed may be raised to a 45-degree angle to help keep swelling down at the incision site, and a sling may be provided to help remind you not to raise the arm on the side of the pacemaker above chest height. During the first six weeks after your pacemaker implant, your heart starts forming scar tissue around the lead tip, or tips, which anchors the lead in place. Until this occurs, raising the arm above your head could pull the lead out of position, requiring another visit to the procedure room.

Before you leave the hospital, you will probably receive a visit from the nurse educator. Most hospitals have a nurse who will give you instructions on how to care for your wound at home, help you schedule your first follow-up appointment at your physician's office, and show you your pacemaker instructions manual and temporary ID card. It is important that you carry your temporary identification card with you until your permanent card arrives at your home. This card is very helpful if you visit an emergency room, or if you change doctors. It contains information on your pacemaker that will allow your doctor to contact the correct company to evaluate your pacemaker, in a timely manner.

When you go to your doctor's office for your first follow-up appointment, the nurse or pacemaker technician will tell you about the frequency of pacemaker follow-ups, check your pacemaker, and give you information on phone checks or remote follow-ups. Most of the pacemaker companies have the capability, or are close to having the capability, for a nurse or pacemaker technician to view the information from your pacemaker while you are at home. However, if you use remote monitoring, you will still have to make office visits to have changes made to your pacemaker.

After the information is collected, your doctor will review the results, make any necessary changes, and then answer any of your questions.

NOTES

CHAPTER 13
ICDs (Implantable Cardiac Defibrillators)

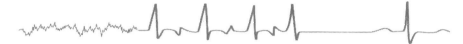

Many of you have seen medical shows where the patient is dying and the doctor rips open the patient's shirt and grabs the paddles, rubbing them together while yelling "Charge to 360"! Then the patient's body jumps as the doctor delivers energy from the defibrillator and, miraculously, the patient comes back to life. Others of you have experienced being defibrillated, or have seen or heard of a relative or friend who was shocked back to life. It does not matter whether the situation is true or fictional, the message is this: if a deadly arrhythmia occurs and the patient can be converted to a normal rhythm quickly, a life can be saved. This is why implantable cardiac defibrillators were developed in the early 1970's.

The first implantable cardiac defibrillators were about the size of a piece of toast and required open-heart surgery to sew defibrillator patches on the heart. (*Figure 23*) The generator was placed in the abdomen, just below the ribcage, with the patch connectors tunneled through the generator pocket. These devices relied only on heart rate to determine if a shock would be delivered. If the heart rate was programmed at 160 beats per minute and you were exercising, you could get an inappropriate shock. Atrial fibrillation presented another problem, because you could be sitting in a chair when atrial fibrillation started, and if your heart rate reached above 160

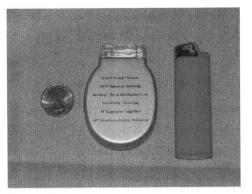

Above, the defibrillator is larger than a pacemaker to accommodate the technology needed to perform the duties of a defibrillator, as well as those of a pacemaker.

Figure 23

beats per minute, you would get shocked. Yet another problem identified with the first defibrillators was that sometimes when a shock was delivered, the heart stopped beating completely. In this instance, cardiopulmonary resuscitation (CPR) would need to be performed until a temporary pace making wire could be placed, or the heart began beating on its own. If this happened, or if the patient also had a bradycardia, or a slow heart rate, a pacemaker system would also be implanted in the left or right upper chest. Over the years, the size of the defibrillator has decreased to smaller than the size of a package of cigarettes, and they all have pacing capabilities. Because of the smaller size of the generator and development of defibrillator leads (the leads that go inside the heart), (*Figure 24*) the defibrillator system is generally implanted in the upper chest.

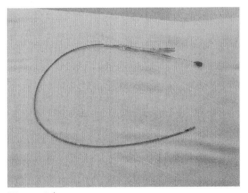

The defibrillator lead is larger than a pacemaker lead, with three connector pins, instead of one for a pacemaker. The other two are for the shocking coils, which can be seen at the middle of the lead and towards the tip of the lead. Having these coils allows the doctor to program the defibrillator for the best chance of a return to normal rhythm, once a deadly arrhythmia occurs. This is the right ventricular lead.

Figure 24

Before we continue, you should understand the basic concept of defibrillation. In a normal heart, an electrical impulse is initiated in the sinoatrial node, spreads uniformly around the atrium, meeting at the atrioventricular node, spreading to the ventricle, and the heart squeezes. When ventricular fibrillation occurs, all the heart cells fire in an erratic manner, causing very fast heart rates that make the heart quiver. When the heart quivers, no blood is pushed out to the body, causing syncope, or passing out, and eventually death. When a person is externally defibrillated, using the paddles, energy greater than the heart cells is sent from one

paddle to the other, forming a wave of energy across the heart. The idea is to fire all the heart cells at one time, and when they recover, they will start to beat uniformly again. This is called a monophasic waveform, or shock, wherein the waveform only goes in one direction, and it is very successful in converting patients' hearts to a normal rhythm, which is the reason the first implantable cardiac defibrillators used this form of technology. Many of the patients requiring defibrillation needed more than one shock to return their hearts to a normal rhythm. In search of the reason why, researchers found that heart cells have a period after being stimulated (shocked) that no amount of energy would reset them. However, once the cell recovered, it would initiate fibrillation all over again. During the 1980's and early 1990's, a biphasic, or two-directional, shock or waveform was developed and refined. When the shock is initiated, it goes in one direction, and midway during the delivery of the energy, it switches, or reverses direction, resetting the cells that were not reset in the first direction. This technology has allowed lower energy to be used for a successful return to normal heart rhythm. This development was excellent for the implantable defibrillator, by using less energy and fewer shocks from the generator battery; the life of the generator was extended. In fact, this technology is so successful that most of the manufacturers of external defibrillators have changed to using the biphasic technology. At this point, I want you to understand that having an implantable defibrillator gives you the greatest chance of surviving a deadly arrhythmia, but it will not keep you from dying if it is your time to go.

The deadly arrhythmias are ventricular fibrillation and ventricular tachycardia (VT). As mentioned earlier, ventricular fibrillation is an erratic, very fast heart rhythm that makes the heart quiver, allowing little or no blood to flow to the body, and, if untreated, leads to death. Ventricular tachycardia can be monomorphic or polymorphic (stable or unstable). Monomorphic

VT comes from one site, whereas, polymorphic VT comes from many sites. Both can be stable or unstable: stable referring to tolerating the increased heart rate and lowered blood pressure and oxygen saturation, and unstable meaning not tolerating these changes and requiring some form of therapy. There are national as well as international guidelines for receiving an implantable cardiac defibrillator, and if your doctor has recommended one, your symptoms fall under these guidelines.

There are three types of defibrillator systems: single-chamber, dual-chamber, and biventricular. The single-chamber system consists of the generator and a defibrillator lead placed in the right ventricle. This system is generally used in patients who have survived a cardiac event, are at risk for another cardiac event, or have need of a pacemaker/defibrillator, and have atrial fibrillation. A dual-chamber defibrillator system includes a generator, a right atrial pacemaker lead, and a defibrillator lead for the right ventricle, and is indicated for patients who have the need for a defibrillator as well as to pace in both the atrium and ventricle. A biventricular defibrillator system entails a generator, right atrial pacing lead, right ventricular defibrillator lead, and a left ventricular pacemaker lead. In the case of a patient requiring biventricular pacing capability, but also having atrial fibrillation, the right atrial pacing lead will not be implanted, and a plug will be placed in the atrial port of the connecting header. These defibrillator systems are for the patients with heart failure that require resynchronization therapy, or pacing the left and right ventricles at an interval that will reduce the heart failure symptoms.

The defibrillator lead mentioned above is a dual-purpose lead. One of its functions is to act as a pacemaker lead, carrying electrical impulses to the heart when pacing is needed. The other function is as part of the defibrillation system. With an external defibrillator, the energy from the generator is sent from one paddle to the other, across the heart, which resets the heart cells. In an implantable cardiac defibrillator system, the newer systems have one or two coils placed on the lead in a manner that allows the generator to send energy across the most surface area as possible. In the older systems, the energy could only be sent from the generator to the coils, or patches, whereas, in the newer systems, the generator can send the energy to the coil in the right ventricle, in turn sending the defibrillation energy to the other coil and the generator. These options have given your doctor the opportunity to program your defibrillator in a way that is the most successful and safest for you.

The generator, itself, is larger than a pacemaker, housing a battery, a capacitor that is used to store energy for the defibrillator, and the computer that controls the function of the device. A typical defibrillator generator has all the basic pacemaker capabilities and most, if not all, of the additional parameters, or bells and whistles. The basic parameters for the defibrillator portion of the generator include a number of zones to monitor, therapies in these zones, the progression of these therapies, and specific therapy programming.

A simple "shock box" has only one programmable zone where the heart rate is set, and when it is above the set rate, the device initiates shock therapy. While these devices are sufficient for some patients, they are used so infrequently that most manufacturers, if not all, have ceased producing them. The majority of devices manufactured today have multiple zone configurations. An example of this would be a three-zone device where the first zone would provide therapy if the rhythm was between 140 and 150 beats per minute, the second zone would be programmed from 160 to 190 beats per minute, and the third zone would be therapy for heart rates above 190 beats per minute.

There are four therapies that can be programmed in different zones, but not all four can be programmed in every zone. First, a monitor zone can be programmed to collect information and store electrograms when the heart rate reaches, as in our example above, the 140-160 zone, but no further action is taken when the heart rate is in this zone. Your doctor would not want this option in the third zone (the defibrillation zone), as heart rates this high need to be converted back to normal quickly. The second therapy is ATP (antitachycardia pacing). The idea behind ATP is that if the heart is paced faster than the ventricular tachycardia rate, and then it suddenly stops, the heart cells would reset without defibrillation being required. The third therapy is cardioversion. Cardioversion is a synchronized, or timed, shock to avoid delivering the energy during a vulnerable period of the electrical impulse, which could deteriorate the rhythm to ventricular fibrillation. The fourth, and final, type of therapy is defibrillation. Here, the energy is delivered as soon as it is available without regard to the timing of the electrical impulse.

Each zone has a certain number of therapies that can be delivered before therapies from the next zone are initiated. Of course, if the zone is programmed to monitor, only, no other therapies are delivered until the heart rate reaches the next heart rate zone. Also, therapies must progress from the least aggressive to the most aggressive, which means that antitachycardia pacing therapy cannot be programmed if the therapy before it is a cardioversion therapy. The next therapy could be a cardioversion with the same energy or higher or a defibrillation therapy.

Each therapy has programmable parameters, some more than others. In the monitor, only, therapy, programming the heart rate is generally the only programming available. In antitachycardia pacing, it allows the most programmable parameters of any of the other therapies, such as how many paced beats are in the pacing train, how many pacing trains to run before moving to the next therapy, should one extra beat be added with each successive pacing train, the rate the pacing train should pace, and any adjustment within the pacing train. ATP therapy allows the most opportunity for a painless conversion from ventricular tachycardia to a normal rhythm before defibrillation begins. In the defibrillation zone, only two parameters are programmable: the heart rate at which your rhythm is considered ventricular fibrillation, and the amount of energy delivered with each shock within this zone. Doctors' views vary in their programming of this zone. Some program the first shock at the defibrillation threshold, some set it a little higher, and some use a tiered therapy, but most set the final therapies at the device's maximum output. The defibrillation threshold, also called DFT, is determined during testing of the device, and is the lowest amount of energy that successfully terminates an arrhythmia.

Beyond the basic programming capabilities that all defibrillators have, the manufacturers set themselves apart with advanced programming capabilities. Some of these include an alert to inform you that something may be wrong with the system, or the battery is nearing replacement indications. There could be in-depth histograms that allow your doctor to see what the device is seeing and providing information used to "fine tune" your system to your individual need. Algorithms allow the device to discriminate between atrial fibrillation and ventricular fibrillation, thus, reducing inappropriate shocks. In the biventricular defibrillator systems most of the manufacturers are developing, one company already has an algorithm to recommend the best timing intervals during pacing, which provides the most efficient heart function. This algorithm takes approximately 90 seconds to determine these values, where the previously used method required 1 to 2 hours. Your doctor's goal is to implant a defibrillator system that allows you to live a life as close to normal as possible while protecting you from fatal arrhythmias.

The defibrillator system implant is very similar to a pacemaker system implant in that all of the instruments used are the same: The patient is sterilely draped for the procedure in a similar manner; the pocket for the generator is formed the same way (although a little larger due to the generator size), access for lead placement mimics that for a pacemaker; and testing the defibrillator lead measurements is accomplished in the same fashion. The difference between a pacemaker system and a defibrillator system implant is that the defibrillator function of the device needs to be tested before completing the procedure.

In certain circumstances, defibrillator function testing will not be performed, such as if the patient is pregnant, which protects the baby, or if your doctor feels that you are too ill. If this is the case, once the baby is born, or once you are in better health, you will return to the procedure room to have the testing performed. The vast majority of patients have their devices tested during the initial implant procedure. If this is you, and a general anesthesia, which is rarely used anymore, is not being applied, your doctor will administer a medication, which is short acting and puts you in a deep sleep while the testing is performed. There are trained personnel continually monitoring your airway and ready to use an external defibrillator, if needed. Once you are in a deep sleep, ventricular fibrillation is induced using the device. During this period, your doctor watches the device reaction to your arrhythmia through the device programmer. Your doctor checks to make sure the device recognizes the arrhythmia, charges the programmed energy, and delivers a shock appropriately returning your heart to a normal rhythm. During this testing, adjustments may need to be made to the device to assure that national or international standards are met for successful device testing. It is important to note that this testing is completed in a controlled environment, with doctors and staff all trained in advanced cardiac life support, so you and your doctor may be confident that the device will work successfully in your normal day-to-day living.

Once all the lead measurements are acceptable and device testing has been completed, your doctor will close the pocket, and a sterile dressing will be applied. After you leave the procedure room, the same post-operative regimen as with a pacemaker will apply: vital signs monitored, chest x-ray performed, and the head of the bed elevated. With all of the post-operative orders complete, you may be released from the hospital the same day, or early the next morning, depending on your doctor's preference. Of course, if you entered the hospital for another reason, you will stay until that situation is resolved.

NOTES

Commonly Asked
Questions

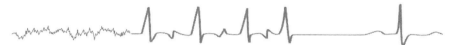

Before I answer some of the most popular questions about the procedures presented in this book, I want you to understand that I am not a cardiologist or an electrophysiologist. My answers are from my experiences over the years, but your doctor may have a different viewpoint, and that viewpoint is what should be followed.

Questions Relating to
All Invasive Procedures

Will I be awake during the procedure?

In most instances, you will be given enough medication that you do not care that you are having the procedure done. The idea is to have you relaxed to the point where you are almost asleep, and you may even fall asleep, but you are able to be aroused, if necessary. In other cases, the doctor may order fewer medications, thinking that medications may hide or mask your arrhythmia if you are too sedated. If you are having your defibrillator tested or are in need of a cardioversion, medications will be used to put you in a deep sleep for a short period of time.

What about my family?

Your family members provide moral as well as spiritual support, which makes each of them an important part of your support system. While your procedure is ongoing, you know what is happening, or do not care, and your family is in a waiting room wondering how the procedure is progressing. Therefore, you should discuss with your doctor how they are to be kept informed. At some procedure labs, the staff will give your family an estimated time for the procedure, and the doctor will meet with them following the procedure. Other labs try to give the family hourly updates, which may be delayed if the procedure is at a critical point. Still other labs will have family members stay in your room where the staff can call the procedure lab for updates. If family members cannot be present for the procedure, a designated family member can be contacted after the procedure, and given the information to pass on to other family members. The message here is to discuss this issue with your doctor before your procedure.

Is my doctor good?

This is something you need to investigate on your own. Family, friends, and acquaintances are a great source of information if they have had experiences with your doctor. Another good source is the internet, looking for things like how long have they been in practice, is this the first place they have worked, where did they attend school, and what research have they published.

What if I am uncomfortable?

As mentioned in the text of the book, there is a staff member responsible for monitoring your vital signs throughout the procedure. This is your contact person, and you should not be shy about expressing your discomfort. The goal of your doctor and staff is to accomplish the procedure in the most efficient and comfortable manner possible. There may be times when medications are withheld for a specific reason, but this should be explained to you prior to the procedure.

What about taking my regular medications?

Most medications can be taken the day of the procedure with sips of water, but medications used to suppress your arrhythmia may be stopped to make testing easier. You should check with your doctor ahead of time as to which medications to take and which medications you should not take.

What if I need to use the restroom during the procedure?

Generally, you will be asked not to eat or drink for 12 hours before your procedure, allowing ample time for your system to clean out. If the situation does arise, using a bedpan is one option. Another for men is a condom catheter. This is worn like a condom but has tubing at the tip that attaches to a collection bag. If you have a history of a weak bladder, a catheter may be inserted prior to the procedure. If this is an option you would like to use, it should be discussed with the doctor or nurse before hospital admission.

What if I do not like my doctor?

Not all patients like the doctors they see, and depending on the size of the city you live in, options are available. If you live in a small community with only one electrophysiologist, you can either "bite your tongue," and live through the experience, or seek a doctor in a nearby town. In larger communities, there are more choices available. You should not feel guilty for changing doctors, however, I suggest you not burn any bridges with your present doctor, as you may want to return to his or her care.

How long is my recovery?

This depends on the procedure. If you have an electrophysiology study or radiofrequency ablation, where only the veins are used for access, it is usually a 2 to 4 hours for recovery, lying fairly flat in bed at the hospital, followed by walking around the unit to make sure the site does not bleed with activity, and 3-7 days of limited activity will allow enough healing enabling you to return to your normal activities.

If arterial access is used, the time in bed is 3 to 6 hours, followed by walking, and 3-7 days of limited activities. For implantable devices, recovery includes 1 to 3 hours in bed, usually with the head of the bed elevated to lessen any swelling, followed by limited use of the arm on the side of the implant for an amount of time designated by the doctor, particularly, if leads were placed. By not raising the arm above chest height, there is less chance that a lead will become dislodged. The doctor-prescribed time for limited activity allows the heart to form scar tissue around the lead tip, anchoring it into position.

What about bruising?

In any invasive procedure, small amounts of bruising are common in the entry site areas, whether in the arm, shoulder, or groin. This is caused by small amounts of blood under the skin and will usually disappear in the first couple of weeks. Lumps (or hematomas) are usually a small complication after a procedure. During the recovery period, hematomas, or a lump caused by incomplete sealing of the vein or artery, may form under the skin. During the recovery period, the sites are checked quite frequently, and if a hematoma is forming, additional pressure will be applied to the site, which serves to stop the bleeding as well as spread the excess blood over a larger area. With a hematoma, you should expect a larger bruise than if one had not formed. The lump will disappear over time as normal activity allows the muscles to break the hematoma into very small particles, which eventually disappear.

If a hematoma forms in the pocket of an implantable device—a loop recorder, pacemaker, or defibrillator, direct pressure will be applied, followed by placement of a sandbag, or pressure dressing, to keep the hematoma from growing. In some cases, a fair amount of blood forms in the pocket and requires another trip to the procedure room to evacuate, or clean out, the pocket. If you believe a hematoma is forming, or if active bleeding occurs after returning home, apply direct pressure to the site with your fingertips and contact your doctor or local emergency room.

When can I start driving again?

This is a question for your doctor, as they know the procedure you had, and what the state laws dictate.

When can I take a shower?

Generally, doctors recommend taking a sponge bath for the first couple of days. Then if the sites are covered, showers are allowable. Baths are not allowed until after 7 to 10 days, as the doctor does not want any dirty bathwater getting into the healing sites, possibly causing infections.

When can I return to normal sexual activity?

Again, this is something to ask your doctor. Your body requires time to heal, and when you return to normal activity you want to be particularly aware if any swelling or bleeding occurs.

Can I listen to music?

Each lab and doctor has a view on whether or not music should be allowed during the procedure. Some labs allow you to bring your own player with headphones while others supply you with headphones, and will play your request from their music selections. Some labs will listen to music the staff enjoys or play music the doctor requests, and there are labs where no music is allowed. If music is important to you, ask your doctor ahead of time about any music restrictions.

Questions About Implantable Devices

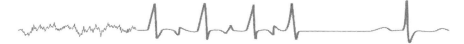

Will I feel the shock?

During defibrillator testing, medications are administered to put you into a short, deep sleep, and you should not feel or remember the shock or shocks. If multiple test shocks need to be performed, additional doses of the medication may be administered until testing has been completed. Once you and your defibrillator are out on your own, you will know when a shock is delivered.

What does a shock feel like?

I can only share what others have told me: "It's like getting kicked in the chest by a mule." "It's like someone punched me in the chest." "It's like someone threw a baseball into my chest." "I knew I had been shocked." "It dropped me to my knees." I have also heard "I didn't know it went off." If your defibrillator is functioning properly, the short time that the pain lasts is better than dying.

After how many shocks should I call the doctor or go to the emergency room?

While even one shock will alarm you, you must understand that this is why you chose to have the defibrillator implanted. You can call your doctor's office or contact the on-call doctor, if after office hours, for advice. The advice is usually to come to the office the following day to have the device evaluated, or to transmit data if you have remote monitoring capabilities with your device. If any programming changes need to be made, an doctor's office visit will be required.

If you receive multiple shocks, you may be advised to go to the emergency room, where a company representative can evaluate your device, if your doctor is not immediately available. At this time, adjustments can be made to the device, if needed, and medications may be reviewed and adjusted, with the consent or recommendation of your doctor. Again, be sure to ask your doctor prior to the procedure, so you have the answer if you need it.

Will my device keep me alive?

Your pacemaker is a machine that puts out an electrical impulse at a predetermined interval. When the heart responds to this impulse, a heartbeat is the result, and if it does not, a skipped beat is the result. This is why the pacemaker is evaluated on a regular basis. During evaluation, a minimal amount of energy to produce a reaction is determined and the device is programmed to two to three times this value to assure that an adequate impulse is created with each beat. In the case of pacemakers with automatic testing, if an impulse is sent and there is no response, the device quickly sends another impulse at a higher energy to assure a heartbeat. In these cases, yes, the pacemaker will keep you alive, but if your heart is so sick that it does not respond to the highest energy that the pacemaker can produce, then death occurs.

With defibrillators, the pacemaker function is the same as above, and the therapies it delivers determine whether or not you survive. This machine is programmed to give you therapies when arrhythmia is detected, and as soon as the arrhythmia is converted to a normal rhythm, it stops delivering therapies. In the case of a very sick heart, all the therapies can be delivered and the arrhythmia can continue, which again will result in death.

The bottom line is that pacemakers and defibrillators provide an excellent therapy for people with electrical problems, but if your heart is too sick, they will not keep you alive.

Will my device be noticeable?

Pacemakers and defibrillators have become smaller over the years, but depending on your body type, it may or may not be visible. In a person with very little body fat, even the smallest pacemaker will be visible. Those with normal body fat may not see the pacemaker, and those with extra body fat may not see a defibrillator. In cases where the look is important, these devices may be placed under the chest muscle, or, in women, a pocket may be formed so that the breast hides their device.

How often does my device need to be checked?

At your first visit to the doctor's office after your device implant, the doctor or nurse will inform you of the schedule, and will set your next appointment before you leave the office that day.

When does my pacemaker or defibrillator need to be replaced?

Each device has some indicators that allow your doctor to know when it is time to replace the generator. It may be the rate the pacemaker paces when a magnet is placed over it, or the battery voltage remaining in either the pacemaker or defibrillator, and in a defibrillator, the amount of time it takes to charge for a shock. There are three stages of a device lifetime: the first is the beginning of life (BOL). The second is elective replacement indicators (ERI). The third is end of life (EOL).

Beginning of life is from the time the device is implanted until it nears elective replacement indication. At each follow-up appointment, these values are evaluated, and as your device nears ERI, your follow-ups will be more frequent, which allows the doctor to help you get the most time out of your device before replacing it. Once the device reaches ERI, your doctor knows that there is anywhere from two weeks to three months before reaching the end of life, and you can be scheduled to have the device changed. If the device reaches end of life, this does not mean it stops working. Rather, it means the device function can be unpredictable. At this point, the device will generally shut down all the bells and whistles that were programmed, and it will function in a very, very basic way.

What does a replacement involve?

A generator replacement involves almost everything your initial implant procedure did, with the exception of putting leads in. The doctor will expose and remove your generator and the leads will be tested. If the lead values are good, a new generator will be connected and the pocket will be closed, with a sterile dressing applied. In a defibrillator generator change, the leads will be evaluated, the new device will be connected, and you will be put into a short, deep sleep while the defibrillator portion of your device is tested. Once all the testing is completed, the pocket will be closed and a sterile dressing will be applied. Normally, a generator change is an outpatient procedure, and once a short recovery period is completed, you will be released from the hospital.

How do I know my pacemaker or my defibrillator is working?

Most of the time you will not, except that you will not experience the symptoms that warranted your getting a device. There have been occasions when patients have told me that they can tell the difference between when the pacemaker is pacing, and when it is not, however, this is just an awareness and not anything alarming. With a defibrillator, the only time you will notice that it is working is if you receive a shock, and if it is functioning appropriately, you should experience some symptoms before receiving this therapy.

Who makes the best pacemaker or defibrillator?

With all being told, all device manufacturers have good devices; otherwise, the Food and Drug Administration (FDA) would not allow them to be sold in the United States, and the same goes for governing bodies in other countries. The items that set one device apart from another are the special features that are available. Your doctor has a thorough knowledge of these devices and recommends the one thought to provide you with the best outcome.

How long will my device last?

This depends on many factors, including how often it is used, what bells and whistles are programmed, and, with defibrillators, how many times it has charged or delivered a shock. Each company has a warranty on their devices, and researching each company and its products something you may wish to do prior to your procedure.

What if it does not last to the warranty time?

As an example, let us say your device has a 5-year warranty, and your doctor tells you it needs to be replaced at 3 years. If the device functioned within normal limits, the manufacturer would supply credit for the full amount of the device, or prorate credit depending on the warranty. Also, there is usually some rebate for your unreimbursed medical costs. Each manufacturer's goal is to supply the medical community with the very best product, but as these are computers run with batteries, there can be situations that arise. If your device needs to be replaced during the warranty period, you should investigate how much money can be put toward the replacement device.

When will the stitches be removed?

Generally between 7 and 10 days, but ask your doctor.

What needs to be done if I have to schedule surgery?

Most surgeries use electrocautery to control bleeding, and the noise this creates can be seen by a pacemaker as your heart rate, telling the pacemaker not to pace, or as an arrhythmia by a defibrillator, telling it to provide therapy. This is why it is important to let your surgeon know you have a device. The surgeon's office can contact your pacemaker or defibrillator doctor to discuss how to proceed with the surgery safely.

What if I don't get my ID card?

Before you leave the hospital, you should receive a booklet on your device and a temporary ID card. If you do not, ask the nurse before you leave. Within the next 30 days, you should receive a laminated permanent ID card. You should carry this with you at all times, as it advises others who need to know about your device any pertinent information necessary. If you do not receive your permanent card within 30 days, call your doctor's office and they will contact the manufacturing company to get you one.

Will a microwave oven affect my device?

No. Years ago, it could have, but both microwave ovens and new devices have better insulation where it has become a non-factor.

Will my cell phone affect my device?

There is little chance your cell phone will affect your device, but manufacturers suggest that you keep the phone at least 6 inches from the device.

What if . . . effects my device?

There are many electrical devices that can effect pacemakers and defibrillators. If you have questions regarding the specific device, you should contact the technical support for the manufacturing company at the 800-number provided on your ID card, and it can provide you with this information.

Can I have an MRI another doctor recommended?

Magnetic resonance imaging (MRI) uses large, very powerful magnets to create images, and, as such, it is generally not an acceptable procedure for people with pacemakers or defibrillators. If another doctor recommends an MRI, he should contact your pacemaker or defibrillator doctor, and the two should discuss how to proceed. In most cases, other options are available, but if this is the only option, it has been safely done with patients. My experiences with pacemaker patients who had the device checked before the MRI, monitored during the MRI, and checked after the MRI had no complications. An MRI in device patients is an issue in hospitals, because there is little information about the interaction. Some hospitals or imaging centers refuse to do the procedure, while others will but under certain conditions. The issue seems to be heat that is generated at the tip of the leads causing them not to function properly. In general, the generator casing is made from material not adversely affected by the large magnets and is not of concern. As of this writing, a proposed MRI is handled on a case-by-case basis, but manufacturers are working to make this a safe and available test for all patients with devices.

How will my device effect my travel?

There are two things to address if you have a device and want to travel: getting through security and service if needed. If you present your device ID card to the security personnel, they will bypass the walk-through unit and use a wand to clear you. Even if you walk through the scanner, it will not effect your device as it is done so quickly, but the device will probably alarm and you will need the wand anyway. If you are traveling within the United States, the 800 number on your ID card will allow you or the doctor taking care of you to access technical support for your device. If you are traveling out of the country, you should contact technical support in the United States for the closest technical support contact at your destination.

Glossary

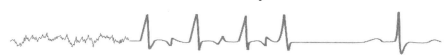

A-H interval The amount of time it takes for an electrical signal to travel from the low right atrium to the his bundle

accessory bypass tract An abnormal electrical pathway that bypasses part of the heart's normal electrical pathway

active fixation leads Leads that attach by deploying a helix that screws into the heart muscle

alert A device function that alerts the patient to abnormal device function through auditory tones or vibrations

antitachycardia pacing Pacing provided by some devices to detect and terminate tachycardias

aorta The largest artery in the body distributing oxygenated blood to all other arteries of the body

aortic valve The valve that separates the left ventricle from the aorta where oxygenated blood is distributed to the body

arteries

The high pressure vessels that deliver oxygenated blood to the body

atria

The upper left and right chambers of the heart

atrial fibrillation

An irregular rapid atrial arrhythmia resulting in erratic and ineffective contraction of the atrium (350 to 600 beats per minute)

atrial flutter (AFL)

An atrial arrhythmia that uses a macroreentrant circuit in the atrium, which usually beats between 250 and 350 beats per minute

atrial tachycardia (AT)

An arrhythmia that arises from the atrium usually between 100-250 beats per minute

atrioventricular nodal reentrant tachycardia (AVNRT)

A supraventricular arrhythmia with dual atrioventricular nodal physiology

atrioventricular

(AV) node

A small concentration of conductive tissue at the junction of the atria and ventricles responsible for initiating electrical impulses in the heart if the sinoatrial node fails, between 40 and 60 beats per minute

biphasic shock

Energy delivered to the heart where the direction of the energy reverses during delivery

biventricular system

A generator and leads in the right atrium, right ventricle and a left ventricular lead placed over the left ventricle through veins of the coronary sinus or attached to the outside of the heart via active fixation

bradycardia | A slow heart rate inappropriate for the patient

capacitor | An electronic circuit component that temporarily stores an electrical charge

cardiologist | A doctor who specializes in the function of the heart

cardioversion | A synchronized shock used to return the heart to a normal rhythm

circulator station | Includes vital sign monitoring equipment, a defibrillator, supplemental oxygen controls and access to the patient

clockwise (CW) flutter | Atrial flutter in which the electrical pathway travels in a clockwise direction

concealed bypass tract | A bypass tract that cannot be identified by a 12-lead EKG

coronary sinus | The largest vein in the heart that returns blood from the heart to the right atrium. It also allows access for evaluation of the electrical system of the heart's left side

counter clockwise
(CCW) flutter | Atrial flutter in which the electrical pathway travels in a counter clockwise direction

defibrillation | An unsynchronized shock used to return the heart to a normal rhythm

defibrillation
threshold (DFT) | The minimum amount of energy required to convert ventricular tachycardia or ventricular fibrillation to normal sinus rhythm

defibrillator generator	A battery, circuitry for programming and a capacitor for producing energy for defibrillation
defibrillator system	A defibrillator generator, defibrillation lead and one or two pacing leads (for dual chamber or biventricular devices)
device pocket	A surgically created cavity for housing the implantable devices
diagnostic electrode catheter	An electrode catheter used to record information from and stimulate the heart
dual chamber system	A generator and leads placed in the right atrium and right ventricle
echocardiography	Recording the position and motion of the heart using ultrasonic waves through the chest wall
electrical pathway	A pathway the electrical impulses of the heart travel
electrical system of the heart	Responsible for initiating the pumping action of the heart. Includes the sinoatrial node, atrioventricular node and bundle branches
electrogram	An electrical representation of the heart's activity
electrophysiologic study (EPS)	An evaluation of the heart's electrical system through the use of recordings and electrical stimulation to expose any arrhythmias
electrophysiologist	A cardiologist who specializes in the electrical system of the human heart

general anesthesia   A state of unconsciousness without pain sensation throughout the entire body

heart block   A disruption of electrical impulses through the atrioventricular conduction system

heart catheterization   An invasive procedure used to monitor the heart function or visualize the veins or arteries of the heart

heart failure   A condition in which the heart is unable to pump its required amount of blood

histogram   A diagnostic feature that records all activities of the device to be reviewed at follow-up appointments

Holter monitor   An ambulatory monitor used to record arrhythmic events usually in a 24-hour period

invasive procedure   Any procedure using surgical incision or venous/arterial puncture for access to the body

isthmus   An area of heart tissue between the tricuspid valve and inferior vena cava

King of Hearts   An ambulatory monitor used to record arrhythmic events usually for one to thirty days

lead impedance   The opposition to a pacing stimulus

loop recorder   A patient triggered event recorder for patients with infrequent arrhythmic events

macro-reentrant circuit   A pathway in which the impulses travel through a large area of tissue

mapping system   A recording system that uses a catheter in the heart chamber or patches on the outside of the chest to create a virtual 3-D image of

	the chamber, useful in diagnosis and therapy of arrhythmias
maze procedure	A surgical procedure for atrial fibrillation during which time the left and right atria are opened and incisions are made in a checker board fashion, and then the atria are sewn closed. The left and right atrial appendages are removed and the pulmonary veins are isolated. This procedure prevents abnormal atrial signals from being conducted
micro reentrant circuit	A pathway in which the impulses travel through a small area of tissue
mitral valve	A two cusped valve that regulates blood flow between the left atrium and left ventricle
monomorphic rhythm	A rhythm that originates from one site where each beat resembles the previous beat
monophasic shock	Energy delivered to the heart in one direction
near syncope	The sensation of losing consciousness without actually passing out
neurocardiogenic syncope	Loss of consciousness due to a low blood pressure with or without bradycardia
outflow tract	The area of heart tissue below the pulmonary or aortic valve
output	The electrical output is delivered from a device
pacemaker generator	A battery and circuitry for programming pacemaker functions

pacemaker system	A pacemaker generator and one, two, or three pacing leads
pacing protocols	A series of paced beats at 100, 125, and 150 beats per minute followed by one, two, or three extra stimuli used to initiate an arrhythmia
palpitations	A sensation of rapid or irregular heart beats
paroxysmal atrial fibrillation	Atrial fibrillation that terminates without the need of cardioversion
passive fixation leads	Leads with tines at the tip that are inserted into the mesh network of tissue in the atria and ventricles
peel away sheath	A small plastic tube used to introduce a pacing or defibrillator lead into the body, and then, it is peeled away leaving the lead in place
permanent atrial fibrillation	Atrial fibrillation that cannot be terminated with drug therapy or electrical cardioversion
persistent atrial fibrillation	Atrial fibrillation that requires the use of drugs or electrical cardioversion to terminate
polymorphic rhythm	a rhythm that originates from multiple sites within a heart chamber where each beat may or may not resemble the previous beat
preventricular contractions (PVCs)	An early heart beat in the ventricle that can give the sensation of a hard heart beat

procedure station	Includes the patient table, x-ray equipment and controls, monitors and equipment table
pulmonary valve	The valve that separates the right ventricle from the pulmonary artery which sends deoxygenated blood to the lungs
pulmonary vein isolation (PVI)	An ablative procedure where the four pulmonary veins in the left atrium are electrically isolated, allowing no abnormal signals to conduct
radiofrequency ablation (RFA)	Destruction of tissue causing an arrhythmia through the use of a radiofrequency generator and electrode catheter
radiofrequency ablation catheter	An electrode catheter with a large electrode tip used to deliver energy to destroy tissue causing an arrhythmia
recording station	Includes recording equipment, stimulator, RF generator and slave screens for x-ray monitors
retrograde conduction	Electrical conduction from the ventricle to the atrium
sensitivity	A programmable function of the device that allows the system to see the heart's own beats and to react if one is not present
sensor	A function of the device that allows it to adjust heart rate to the level of activity
septum	A dividing wall of tissue that separates the atria and ventricles

sheath	A small plastic tube with or without a hemostatic valve to prevent backbleeding that can be placed in an artery or vein
sick sinus syndrome	Refer to sinus node dysfunction
single chamber system	A generator and a lead placed in the right atrium or right ventricle
sinoatrial (SA) node	The natural pacemaker of the heart that initiates electrical impulses faster than any other heart cells, between 60 and 100 beats per minute
sinus node dysfunction	Abnormalities in sinus node activity or conduction causing slower, irregular heart rates or tachycardia
stable rhythm	Regular rhythm that maintains stable vital signs
stimulator	A device that uses electrical current to initiate a heart beat
stored electrogram	A programmable function of a device to record short, specific representations of abnormal heart function
stress testing	A diagnostic procedure that determines the body's response to physical exertion while monitoring the patient's vital signs
supraventricular tachycardia (SVT)	An arrhythmia that originates above the ventricles
syncope	Loss of consciousness
tachycardia	Abnormally fast heart rate, usually above 100 beats per minute
threshold	The minimum level of stimulation needed to evoke a response from the heart

tilt table test	A technique used to provoke neurocardiogenic syncope where the patient's heart rate and blood pressure are monitored while tilted to an 80 degree angle
transeptal approach	A procedure which gains left heart access from the venous system by going through the intra atrial septum
tricuspid valve	A three cusped valve that regulates blood flow between the right atrium and right ventricle
12-lead EKG	An electrical recording of the heart representing each heart beat in twelve different vectors
unstable rhythm	An irregular rhythm where vital signs become unstable and may require intervention
veins	The low pressure vessels that return deoxygenated blood through the heart to the lungs to collect oxygen
ventricular apex	The lowest point in the ventricle
ventricular fibrillation	An arrhythmia where the ventricles quiver in an uncoordinated fashion not allowing enough blood flow to sustain life
ventricular tachycardia	A fast circuit (greater than 120 beats per minute) contained in the ventricles
ventricles	The lower left and right chambers of the heart
voltage doubler	A voltage multiplier that allows twice the voltage normally supplied by the circuit
Wolff Parkinson White syndrome	An accessory bypass tract visible on a 12-lead EKG

Proof

Made in the USA
Charleston, SC
12 December 2011